Trauma Vivas for the FRCS (Tr & Orth)

A Case-Based Approach

T0313386

Trauma Vivas for the FRCS (Tr & Orth)

A Case-Based Approach

Raymond Anakwe
Scott Middleton

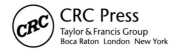

CRC Press
Taylor & Francis Group
Boca Raton London New York

CRC Press is an imprint of the
Taylor & Francis Group, an **informa** business

CRC Press
Taylor & Francis Group
6000 Broken Sound Parkway NW, Suite 300
Boca Raton, FL 33487-2742

© 2018 by Taylor & Francis Group, LLC
CRC Press is an imprint of Taylor & Francis Group, an Informa business

No claim to original U.S. Government works

Printed on acid-free paper

International Standard Book Number-13: 978-1-4987-8097-1 (Paperback); 978-1-1380-6203-0 (Hardback)

Visit the Taylor & Francis Web site at
http://www.taylorandfrancis.com

and the CRC Press Web site at
http://www.crcpress.com

CONTENTS

Preface   ix
Authors   xi

Section I: Lower Limb and Pelvic Trauma

1   Talus Fracture   3
2   Lisfranc Injury   7
3   Subtalar Dislocation   11
4   Calcaneal Fracture   13
5   Triplane Fracture   17
6   Ankle Fracture   21
7   Ankle Fracture   23
8   Infected Ankle   25
9   Pilon Fracture   27
10   Midshaft Diaphyseal Tibia Fracture   33
11   Compartment Syndrome   37
12   Tibial Diaphyseal Fracture (Proximal)   41
13   Mangled Extremity   43
14   Tibial Plateau Fracture   47
15   Knee Dislocation   51
16   Floating Knee   55
17   Distal Femoral Fracture   57
18   Young Femoral Fracture   59
19   Ipsilateral Femoral Neck and Shaft Fracture   63
20   Hip Fracture (Subtrochanteric)   65
21   Pathological Fracture   67
22   Intracapsular Hip Fracture Young Patient   71
23   Hip Fracture   75
24   Periprosthetic Fracture   79
25   Posterior Dislocation of the Hip   81
26   Acetabulum Fracture   83
27   Pelvic Fracture   87
28   Pelvic Fracture   89

Section II: Spine and Upper Limb Trauma

29   Bilateral Cervical Facet Dislocation   95
30   Thoracolumbar Spine Injury   97
31   Proximal Humerus Fracture   99

32	Proximal Humerus Fracture	101
33	Greater Tuberosity Fracture	103
34	Anterior Shoulder Dislocation	105
35	Posterior Dislocation of Shoulder	109
36	Clavicle Fracture	113
37	Acromioclavicular Joint Injury	115
38	Midshaft Humerus Fracture	117
39	Holstein–Lewis Fracture	121
40	Distal Humerus Fracture	123
41	Elbow Dislocation	127
42	Terrible Triad Injury	131
43	Radial Head Fracture	133
44	Olecranon Fracture	135
45	Monteggia Fracture	137
46	Galeazzi Fracture	139
47	Both Bones Forearm Fracture	141
48	Distal Radius Fracture	143
49	Scaphoid Fracture	145
50	Perilunate Dislocation	147
51	Lunate Dislocation	151
52	Fight Bite	153
53	Jersey Finger	155

Section III: General Trauma Principles

54	ATLS	161
55	Open Fracture	165
56	Damage Control Orthopaedics	171
57	Gunshot Injury	173
58	Screws	175
59	Plates	179
60	Nails and External Fixators	181
61	Non-Union	183
62	Non-Accidental Injury	187
63	Osteoporosis	191

Section IV: Surgical Approaches

64	Deltopectoral Approach	195
65	Anterior Approach to Humerus	197
66	Anterolateral Approach to Humerus	199

67	Posterior Approach to Distal Humerus	201
68	Anterior/Volar (Henry's) Approach to the Forearm	203
69	Kocher's and Kaplan's Approaches	207
70	Smith–Petersen Approach	209
71	Ilioinguinal Approach	211
72	Posterolateral Approach to Ankle	215
73	Leg Fasciotomy (Two-Incision/Four-Compartment Fasciotomy)	217

Index 219

PREFACE

The trauma viva should not present any surprises for the well-prepared candidate. Trauma forms a key part of orthopaedic training from day one and the examination aims to test the knowledge expected of a new consultant in the generality of trauma. In this respect, the topics likely to be raised can often be predicted and questions are usually presented in the form of a clinical vignette, photograph or an x-ray to initiate discussion. The exact format will vary from examiner to examiner and between candidates but will often start with a straightforward opening question that a safe candidate would be expected to address without difficulty. Subsequent questions may then test the boundaries of knowledge with extra marks for awareness of the literature and current areas of debate. The examiner is looking to have a conversation with a colleague about the range of trauma that may present in everyday practice and to establish the experience and confidence of the trainee in this area.

This text aims to present key issues in a case-based format. As ever, there are often several ways to address any problem. One safe and accepted way is presented for the cases here. At a basic level, the candidate should be able to recognise the injury, potential problems and complications and explain the rationale and evidence behind their management. The viva examination is not the ideal time to describe an operation that you have never seen or read about. Describing what you have seen and done in your training will usually be sufficient as long as it represents safe practice and recognises that certain areas of treatment may be contentious, debated or require particular expertise.

As always, it is important to listen to the question. The examiner will often steer the discussion to cover specific areas in the allotted time but it is useful to demonstrate that you recognise a particular injury as a 'high-energy injury', that you are familiar with established resuscitation systems such as the ATLS system, that you recognise the potential for associated injuries in severely injured patients and that there may be a variety of options for treatment. Once it is clear that this is routine for the candidate, the examiner will often move you on. If asked what you would do, answer the question succinctly but briefly say why or what factors would make you choose this treatment option.

Keep calm. Stay safe. Good luck!

AUTHORS

Raymond Anakwe is a military and fellowship-trained trauma and orthopaedic surgeon working as a consultant at St Mary's Hospital and Imperial College Hospital NHS Trust in London. He has published widely in trauma surgery and elective orthopaedics and has presented at international conferences all over the world. He is a surgical trainer and is responsible for medical education for surgeons at Imperial College Hospital NHS Trust. Dr Anakwe has a special interest in surgery of the hand, wrist and elbow, as well as trauma care developed during his training in the Edinburgh Trauma Unit and over his 20 years of experience in the British Army with tours in Iraq, Afghanistan and Kosovo. He has a diploma in the medical care of catastrophes and previously won the highly sought-after Winston Churchill Fellowship, visiting major trauma centres throughout the United States. He was also awarded a British Orthopaedic Association travelling fellowship to visit and work at the renowned Chris Hani Baragwanath Hospital in Johannesburg.

Scott Middleton is a trauma and orthopaedic registrar at the Edinburgh Orthopaedic Trauma Unit and a Surgical Education Fellow at the Imperial College Healthcare NHS Trust in London. He is widely published in the orthopaedic literature with more than 20 publications, and review articles for the *British Medical Journal* (*BMJ*) and the *Journal of the American Medical Association* (*JAMA*). He has previously worked on similar projects in his role as the director of medical publishing for EduSurg, creating passthemrcs.co.uk, a highly successful website aimed at trainees about to sit the MRCS part B, which has more than 3000 users. Middleton co-authored a chapter titled 'Assessment of the Multiply Injured Patient' in the newly published *Oxford Textbook of the Fundamentals of Surgery* and has a special interest in trauma surgery both clinically and academically. Middleton is also a quality improvement trainee associate at NHS Education for Scotland, as well as a clinical tutor associate at the University of Edinburgh.

Section I
LOWER LIMB AND PELVIC TRAUMA

1

TALUS FRACTURE

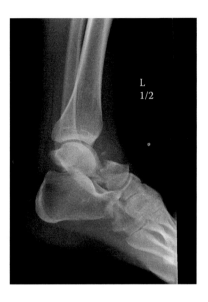

1. **Can you describe the radiograph?**

   This is a lateral radiograph of the left ankle showing a displaced talar neck fracture. The subtalar joint is clearly dislocated, but the tibiotalar and talonavicular joints are congruent. This therefore represents a Hawkins type II fracture.

2. **How are these injuries classified, and what is the importance of the classification system?**

   These are described as follows, according to the Hawkins classification. The importance is that the grade of injury can predict subsequent risk of developing AVN.

   Type I – Undisplaced neck fracture: 10% risk

   Type II – Displaced neck fracture with subluxation/dislocation of the subtalar joint: 30–60% risk

   Type III – Displaced neck fracture with subluxation/dislocation of the subtalar and tibiotalar joints: 60–90% risk

   Type IV – Displaced neck fracture with subluxation/dislocation of the subtalar, tibiotalar and talonavicular joints: Up to 100% risk

3. **What is the typical mechanism of injury?**

   The classical mechanism is an axial load to the dorsiflexed foot. This commonly occurs in road traffic accidents whereby the load from the pedal forces the talar neck against the anterior tibial plafond.

4. **How would you initially manage this injury?**

   This is a high-energy injury and should therefore be managed in the emergency department with concurrent assessment and resuscitation as per ATLS guidelines.

I would assess the neurovascular status of the limb and perform a circumferential examination of the skin to look for any signs of an open fracture. I would ensure the patient had satisfactory analgesia and place the patient in a below knee backslab prior to obtaining a CT scan.

5. How would you definitively manage this fracture?

I would treat this displaced talar neck fracture with open reduction and internal fixation. I would approach this using an anterolateral incision and possibly an additional anteromedial incision.

The anterolateral approach involves a longitudinal incision in the line of the fourth metatarsal, centred on the extensor digitorum brevis which directly overlies the subtalar joint and lateral talar neck. The superficial peroneal nerve is at risk here and full-thickness incisions without undermining are imperative. The extensor digitorum brevis is split and retracted, exposing the lateral aspect of the talar neck. Since the majority of fractures on the lateral side are simple compared with comminution on the medial side, a 'cortical key' can be achieved to obtain reduction. If this is not possible, additional access and exposure can be obtained through an additional anteromedial approach.

The additional anteromedial approach involves an incision from the medial malleolus proximally to the base of the first metatarsal distally. The dissection is between the tibialis anterior and tibialis posterior, protecting the saphenous vein. This exposes the medial aspect of the neck and the body, although it may endanger the deltoid branch of the posterior tibial artery, which is often the only remaining supply to the body of the talus. This dual approach can be used when there is difficulty with reduction.

I would debride the subtalar joint to remove any debris and confirm the fracture reduction using image intensification. Once reduced, I would fix the fracture temporarily with K-wires before applying definitive fixation with two cannulated, partially threaded, cancellous screws.

6. What complications would you warn the patient about?

Starting with early complications, these would include wound dehiscence and infection, particularly in open fractures. Compartment syndrome of the foot may complicate this high-energy injury.

Late complications include AVN, secondary OA, delayed union, mal-union and non-union.

Mal-union typically produces a varus deformity of the hindfoot due to compression of the comminuted medial portion and subsequent loss of length of the medial column of the foot.

7. What is the blood supply to the talus?

The talus has a complicated blood supply which is formed by three main arteries:

1. Posteror tibial artery, leading to:
    a. Artery of the tarsal canal (main supply to the body)
    b. Deltoid branch (may be the only remaining supply in a displaced neck fracture)
2. Dorsalis pedis artery (supplies the talar head and neck)
3. Peroneal artery, leading to:
    Artery of the tarsal sinus

8. **What is Hawkins sign?**

This is the presence of a subchondral lucency in the talar dome, best seen at the superior aspect of the talar body on an AP radiograph, approximately 2 months following the injury. The appearance of decreased subchondral bone density indicates that there is sufficient vascular supply to the bone to allow normal disuse osteopenia (due to subchondral resorption) to occur.

2

LISFRANC INJURY

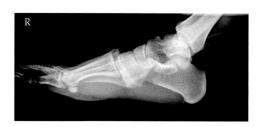

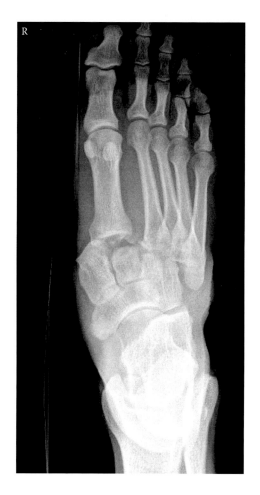

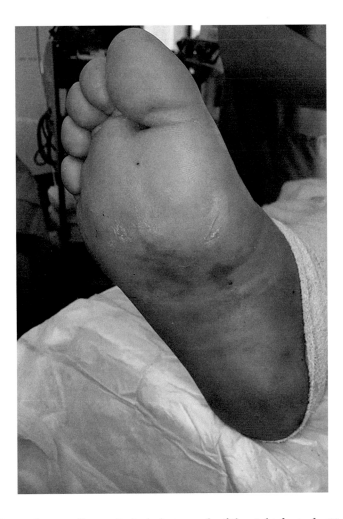

These are radiographs as well as a clinical photograph of the right foot of a 68-year-old man who stumbled down some stairs, injuring his right foot.

1. **Describe these radiographs.**

   These are radiographs of the right foot. They show widening between the first and second metatarsals. There is a fracture at the base of the second metatarsal. This represents a Lisfranc injury.

2. **Describe the clinical photograph and what findings you would expect on examination.**

   The photograph shows the classical finding is of a large medial plantar ecchymosis. Often patients will be unable to weight bear, which is in contrast to a midfoot sprain. Tenderness may be present throughout the whole tarsometatarsal joint region and there may be obvious soft tissue swelling.

3. **What additional imaging may be useful where the diagnosis is unclear and how would you interpret this?**

   I would initially request imaging in the form of anteroposterior, lateral and 30-degree oblique internally rotated plain radiographs of the foot. I would request that these are weight bearing radiographs if this can be tolerated by the patient. The anteroposterior radiograph may show obvious, as in this case, or subtle widening between the first and second metatarsals. A small chip of bone is often evident: 'the fleck sign'. This represents an avulsion from the second metatarsal or the medial cuneiform. Normal alignment on the anteroposterior view is represented by examining the lateral borders of the first and second metatarsals, which should line up with the lateral borders of the medial and middle cuneiforms, respectively. The oblique internally rotated view should also show that the medial border of the fourth metatarsal lines up with the medial border of the cuboid.

On the lateral radiograph, no metatarsal bone should lie more dorsally than the respective tarsal bone.

I would also look for any evidence of fractures in or widening between the cuneiforms. Any abnormalities may all be accentuated on weight bearing radiographs. Computed tomography can be used to image fractures and exclude occult injuries while MR imaging may allow direct visualisation of the Lisfranc ligament itself.

4. How would you manage this patient?
If there is significant soft tissue swelling, I would admit the patient for elevation and regular ice treatment.

This injury represents an unstable articular injury. In the absence of any obvious contraindication I would advise that this patient should be treated operatively.

In an appropriately consented and anaesthetised patient and with a proximal thigh tourniquet, I would make a clinical and radiographic assessment for any instability between the medial and middle cuneiforms. If this is apparent then I would reduce and hold this articulation with a pointed reduction clamp first and then a percutaneous Kirschner wire.

I would use a dual dorsal incision approach. The first incision is based between the first and second metatarsals to address the first and second tarsometatarsal (TMT) joints. This will be centred over the TMT joint area and will allow access to the plane between extensor hallucis longus and extensor hallucis brevis, the latter of which is superficial to the neurovascular bundle. The second incision, if required, is between the third and fourth metatarsals at the same level.

I would inspect and address the second tarsometatarsal joint first. I would reduce the joint and hold this temporarily using an AO reduction clamp before securing this reduction with a 3.5 millimetre cortical lag screw passed from the medial cuneiform (through a separate stab incision) into the base of the second metatarsal, recreating the Lisfranc ligament.

I would then examine the first tarsometatarsal joint for instability. If required, I would reduce and fix this using a 3.5 millimetre cortical lag screw from the first metatarsal into the medial cuneiform.

If required, I would then turn my attention to the third TMTJ, which will be accessed through the second incision. I would stabilise the third ray against the secure second ray by passing a 3.5 millimetre cortical lag screw from the base of the third metatarsal into the lateral cuneiform.

Fixation of the medial TMT joints will often lead to indirect reduction of the fourth and fifth TMT joints. I would examine the lateral two rays for instability using image intensification and, if required, stabilise these rays using 1.6 millimetre K-wires from the respective metatarsals into the cuboid.

I would reassess the foot for intercuneiform instability and, if required, pass a 4.5 millimetre cannulated screw over the K-wire holding the middle and medial cuneiforms.

Postoperatively, I would place the patient in a below knee backslab and would inspect the wounds at 2 weeks and obtain further radiographs. I would advise the patient to remain non-weight bearing on the operated side for 8 weeks.

5. **How might your treatment change in the case of a delayed presentation?**
For presentations up to 6 weeks, I would still consider open reduction and fixation. For older injuries, the results of this treatment are less satisfactory. I would offer a symptomatic patient arthrodesis of the medial three tarsometatarsal joints. This would use the same surgical approach as acute fixation but would necessitate removal of any remaining articular cartilage and stabilisation of the medial three tarsometatarsal joints using lag screws or plates. An extensive delay before presentation may mean that to realign the joints before fusion, soft tissue releases are also required.

FURTHER READING

Dubois-Ferrière V, Lübbeke A, Chowdhary A, Stern R, Dominguez D, Assal M. Clinical outcomes and development of symptomatic osteoarthritis 2 to 24 years after surgical treatment of tarsometatarsal joint complex injuries. *J Bone Joint Surg Am.* 2016 May 4;98(9):713–720.

Eleftheriou KI, Rosenfeld PF, Calder JD. Lisfranc injuries: An update. *Knee Surg Sports Traumatol Arthrosc.* 2013 Jun;21(6):1434–1446.

Lau S, Howells N, Millar M, De Villiers D, Joseph S, Oppy A. Plates, screws, or combination? Radiologic outcomes after Lisfranc fracture dislocation. *J Foot Ankle Surg.* 2016 Apr 12;pii: S1067–2516(16).

3

SUBTALAR DISLOCATION

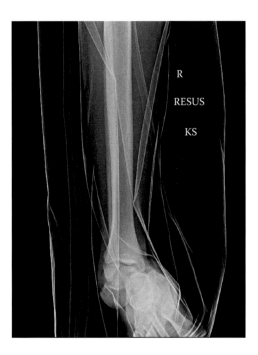

A 28-year-old man is brought to the emergency department after falling from a high wall late in the evening at around 10 p.m. He has a clinically swollen and deformed foot and ankle, and a single radiograph is shown here.

1. **Describe this x-ray.**

    This is an AP radiograph of the tibia, ankle and hindfoot. The view is partially obscured by a plaster or splint. The radiograph shows a medial subtalar dislocation with the calcaneus and the rest of the foot displaced medial to the talus.

2. **This is an isolated injury. Describe your initial management of the patient and this injury.**

    Having treated this patient along ATLS guidelines and established that this is an isolated injury, I would examine the limb carefully, looking to identify any open wounds or threatened skin as a result of the dislocation. I would ensure that the patient had adequate analgesia and make a careful assessment of the neurovascular status. The radiograph does not show any obvious associated fractures, but I would scrutinise it carefully. I would arrange to perform a closed reduction of the dislocation in the emergency department under sedation. I would assess the stability of the reduction, repeat the neurovascular assessment, place the patient in a below knee backslab and confirm the reduction with further radiographs.

3. If it is not possible to achieve a closed reduction, how would you proceed?

In this situation I would make arrangements to take the patient to the operating theatre. I would attempt a closed reduction under formal general anaesthesia, and should this fail, I would undertake this as an open procedure in the operating theatre. If a CT could be arranged urgently then I would arrange it, but I would not allow this to cause delay, especially where there is evidence of vascular injury, threatened skin or soft tissue compromise. In the operating theatre, once consented, positioned and anaesthetised, I would use an anteromedial incision. A closed reduction may be prevented by the talar head becoming buttonholed through the capsule, caught in the extensor retinaculum or impacted into the navicular, causing a mechanical obstruction to reduction. An open approach would allow me to identify and address any of these. I would debride and wash out any wounds and confirm the reduction using image intensification. I would also scrutinise the images for evidence of any associated fractures. I would arrange further imaging with CT after reduction if not already obtained.

4. Describe your plan for definitive management.

Most subtalar dislocations without significant associated fractures are stable after reduction. Treatment in a non-weight bearing below knee cast for 6 weeks is usually sufficient. Where the reduction is unstable as a result of the injury or following debridement, CT may identify additional fractures that should be treated. Where the reduction is unstable as a result of soft tissue injury, I would stabilise the subtalar and talonavicular joints with smooth Steinmann pins augmented with a below knee non-weight bearing plaster cast. I would remove both and commence rehabilitation after 6 weeks.

5. How would you advise the patient as to the likely outcome for this injury and treatment?

These are not common injuries. Fortunately, persistent instability is infrequent. Complications vary and seem to be related to the degree of energy of the injury. Post-traumatic arthritis evident on radiographs is common although the symptomatic effects of these changes may vary. These may be a result of injury to the joint surface, occult fractures or persistent instability. Open fracture dislocations with associated injuries to the nerves, vessels and related tendons (tibial nerve, posterior tibial artery or posterior tibial tendon) have been associated with worse outcomes.

FURTHER READING

Bibbo C, Anderson RB, Davis WH. Injury characteristics and the clinical outcome of subtalar dislocations: A clinical and radiographic analysis of 25 cases. *Foot Ankle Int.* 2003 Feb;24(2):158–163.

Bibbo C, Lin SS, Abidi N, Berberian W, Grossman M, Gebauer G, Behrens FF. Missed and associated injuries after subtalar dislocation: The role of CT. *Foot Ankle Int.* 2001 Apr;22(4):324–328.

Heck BE, Ebraheim NA, Jackson WT. Anatomical considerations of irreducible medial subtalar dislocation. *Foot Ankle Int.* 1996 Feb;17(2):103–106.

4

CALCANEAL FRACTURE

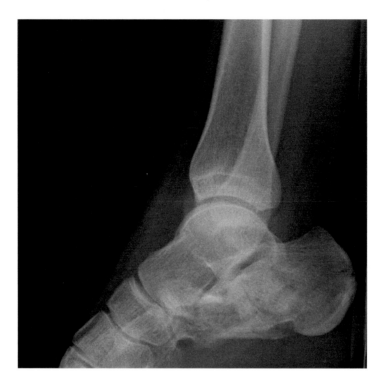

A 35-year-old man is brought to the emergency department after jumping to the ground from a 10-foot wall while being pursued by the police. He complains of bilateral heel pain.

1. **Describe this x-ray.**
   This is a lateral radiograph of the ankle and hindfoot. It shows an intra-articular, displaced and comminuted fracture of the calcaneus with an increased angle of Gissane and a decreased Bohler angle.

2. **With this mechanism of injury, what other injuries might you suspect?**
   This injury has resulted from axial loading. Vertebral fractures, ligamentous injuries around the knee, tibial plateau fractures as well as pilon fractures should be suspected and looked for. Patients may also present with injuries to the contralateral calcaneus.

3. **How would you treat this calcaneus fracture?**
   In making this judgement it would be essential to consider patient factors including general health, diabetes, neuropathy, peripheral vascular disease, smoking status and patient reliability or compliance. It would also be important to consider the personality of the injury. Open wounds, threatened skin, soft tissue swelling and the degree of comminution will all influence management and outcome. Further

imaging in the form of a CT would provide additional information about the fracture pattern, degree of comminution and amenability to fixation of the fracture.

There is some debate about the benefits of surgery however, the evidence for non-operative treatment of displaced fractures is contentious. For this displaced intra-articular fracture, in a suitable patient I would recommend surgery. The aim is to restore the articular surface while restoring calcaneal height, length and heel width. I would give prophylactic antibiotics, position the patient in the lateral position with the foot on a radiolucent table and a thigh tourniquet in place.

I would approach the calcaneus by raising full thickness flaps using a lateral approach centred halfway between the fibular and Achilles tendon and curving anteriorly around the lateral malleolus along the border between the glabrous and non-glabrous skin, keeping the corner angle of the incision greater than 100 degrees. The sural nerve is protected and the lateral calcaneal wall is exposed and lifted out, providing access to the constant medial fragment which bears the sustentaculum tali. I would lever and reduce the constant fragment into position through the fracture and then pass a Steinmann Pin into the calcaneal tuberosity through a separate stab incision adjacent to the Achilles tendon. The Steinmann Pin is used to lever the calcaneal tuberosity into a reduced position and to correct any varus deformity before it is advanced to secure the tuberosity to the constant medial fragment.

The posterior facet articular surface is then reduced, depressed fragments are elevated and the joint surface restored and provisionally held with K-wires before it is fixed definitively with one or more lag screws. I would then replace the lateral wall and secure it with a lateral locking plate and screws. I would perform the procedure using image intensification to allow accurate reduction. I would maintain this patient in a below knee non-weight bearing cast for at least 6 weeks after surgery.

4. What are the complications of surgery, and are there any situations where non-operative management might be preferred?

The immediate complications of surgery include bleeding, malreduction and iatrogenic injury to the cutaneous nerves and peroneal tendons. Open wounds, contused or threatened soft tissues, poor vascular status and diabetes may predispose to wound breakdown, dehiscence and infection. Soft tissue injury and subsequent management strongly influence outcome and fixation may need to be delayed or avoided in some cases. Marked soft tissue swelling should be treated with formal elevation and ice treatment. The wrinkle test is widely used to determine when the soft tissues may be safely tackled, although evidence for this is not strong. Open wounds should be treated with staged debridement, negative pressure dressings, intravenous antibiotic therapy and wound closure or coverage. Smoking has been shown to predispose to non-union, and patients should be encouraged to give it up. In the long term, patients may suffer subtalar arthritis, chronic infection or osteomyelitis, chronic heel pain and complex regional pain syndrome.

Non-operative management is appropriate for undisplaced fractures, minimally displaced extra-articular fractures, anterior process fractures involving less than 25% of the calcaneocuboid joint and patients who are unfit for surgery or where the associated risks are judged to be too high. One randomised control study has suggested that non-operative treatment is appropriate for a broader section of these fractures but this is debated and the study examined a highly selected group of fractures only.

FURTHER READING

Buckley R, Tough S, McCormack R, Pate G, Leighton R, Petrie D, Galpin R. Operative compared with nonoperative treatment of displaced intra-articular calcaneal fractures: A prospective, randomized, controlled multicenter trial. *J Bone Joint Surg Am.* 2002 Oct;84-A(10):1733–1744.

Folk JW, Starr AJ, Early JS. Early wound complications of operative treatment of calcaneus fractures: Analysis of 190 fractures. *J Orthop Trauma.* 1999 Jun–Jul;13(5):369–372.

Griffin D, Parsons N, Shaw E, Kulikov Y, Hutchinson C, Thorogood M, Lamb SE, UK Heel Fracture Trial Investigators. Operative versus non-operative treatment for closed, displaced, intra-articular fractures of the calcaneus: Randomised controlled trial. *BMJ.* 2014 Jul 24;349.

Sanders R, Fortin P, DiPasquale T, Walling A. Operative treatment in 120 displaced intraarticular calcaneal fractures. Results using a prognostic computed tomography scan classification. *Clin Orthop Relat Res.* 1993 May;(290):87–95.

5

TRIPLANE FRACTURE

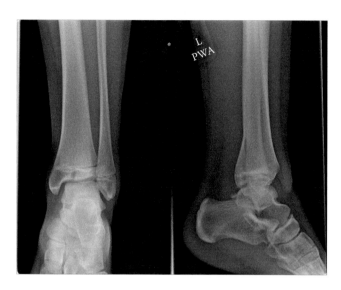

1. Can you describe the radiographs?

These are AP and lateral radiographs of the left ankle in a skeletally immature patient, showing a triplane fracture.

2. Can you describe the fracture in more detail?

Triplane fractures are complex intra-articular injuries with a fracture in all three planes (coronal, axial, saggital), and are the result of an external rotation type injury. The epiphysis is fractured in the saggital plane, and is therefore best visualised on the AP radiograph. The physis itself is disrupted in the axial plane. Finally, the metaphysis is fractured in the coronal plane and the eponymous Thurstan Holland sign/fragment is best seen on the lateral view.

3. At what age do these injuries occur and why?

These injuries are seen in early adolescence, where the physeal fusion starts centrally, then medially and finally extends posterolaterally before finishing with the anterolateral portion.

4. Through which zone of the physis does the fracture occur?

Physeal fractures most commonly occur through the hypertrophic zone. This is the weakest portion of the physis due to the increase in chondrocyte size and subsequent reduction in matrix volume.

5. How would you manage the injury seen in the radiographs?

This is an intra-articular injury which may require open reduction and internal fixation. I would want to assess for an articular step-off with a CT scan, as the radiographs may underestimate the injury. Fractures with displacement <2 mm can be managed conservatively in a below knee, non-weight bearing cast, with vigilant follow-up to observe for displacement.

Fractures with intra-articular displacement require either closed (or open reduction if necessary) in theatre, followed by internal fixation. Closed reduction would consist of reversing the deforming force, and therefore reduce with internal rotation. My preferred choice of fixation would be with two cannulated screws, one in the epiphyseal fragment from medial to lateral and one in the Thurstan Holland fragment from anterior to posterior. I would then place the patient in a below knee plaster of Paris backslab in theatre and instruct the parents and the child to remain non-weight bearing for at least 4 weeks whilst the fracture heals.

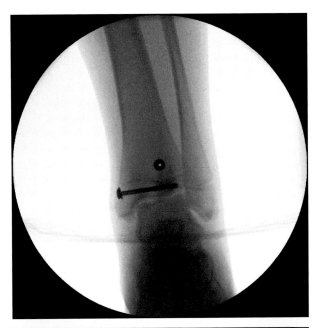

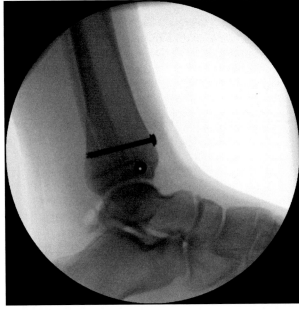

6. **How do these injuries differ from a Tillaux fracture?**

Both the triplane and Tillaux fractures occur in early adolescence. The Tillaux fracture is an avulsion of the Chaput tubercle, where the anterior inferior tibiofibular ligament inserts onto the anterolateral portion of the epiphysis. The Tillaux fracture is intra-articular with a Salter–Harris type III component similar to that seen in the triplane, except that it does not extend into the metaphysis. Both injuries may require reduction and internal fixation if sufficiently displaced.

6

ANKLE FRACTURE

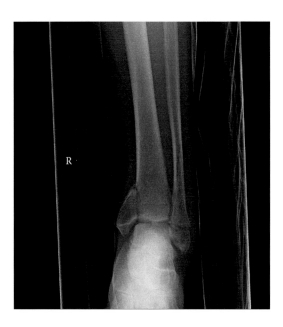

1. **Can you describe the radiograph?**
   This is an AP and lateral radiograph of the left ankle. It shows a bimalleolar ankle fracture.

2. **How would you classify this injury, and how is it best managed definitively?**
   I would use the Lauge–Hansen classification to identify the injury and guide my management. This is a supination–adduction (SAD) type injury. In this case, the joint does appear generally congruent but where there is joint subluxation I would undertake emergent relocation in the emergency department under sedation with a thorough pre- and post-reduction neurovascular assessment. Assuming there is no contraindication to surgery, I would advise surgical management.

   The important point regarding this is recognition of the articular impaction of the tibial plafond. This is best addressed from the medial side first, using the split in the medial malleolus to access the marginal impaction. This is disimpacted and reduced first before the vertical shear type fracture of the medial malleolus is buttressed with a plate. I would then turn my attention to the distal fibula, where I would reduce the fracture through a direct lateral approach and apply a lag screw and neutralisation plate. I would allow the patient to mobilise as able in a below knee cast for a period of 6 weeks before removing the plaster cast.

   I would restrict the weight bearing status of the patient in a below knee cast for a period of 6 weeks before commencing weight bearing due to the intra-articular nature of the injury.

3. **What other types of ankle fracture are identified by the Lauge–Hansen classification system?**

The Lauge–Hansen classification was based on a cadaveric study where the ankle was held in either supination or pronation, and further subdivided by the deforming forces which were applied (adduction, abduction and external rotation). This demonstrated a reliable sequence of injuries which occurred sequentially with increasing force. There are two supination type injuries and two pronation type injuries.

The injury pictured above is a SAD type ankle fracture. This only has two stages. First, there is a transverse avulsion type fracture of the distal fibula or ATFL rupture, followed by a vertical sheer type fracture of the medial malleolus with varying degrees of articular impaction.

The second supination type injury is the most common ankle fracture: The supination–external rotation (SER) type ankle fracture. This has four stages: SER 1 consists of rupture of the AITFL; SER 2 is characterised by the classical oblique fracture of the fibula at the level of the syndesmosis; SER 3 involves the posterior structures with either a rupture of the PITFL or a fracture of the posterior malleolus; SER 4 is the final stage, which involves the medial side with an oblique medial malleolus fracture or rupture of the deep deltoid ligament.

The first of the pronation injuries is the pronation–external rotation (PER) type ankle fracture. This has four stages: PER 1 consists of an oblique medial malleolus fracture or deep deltoid ligament rupture; PER 2 progresses to an AITFL rupture or avulsion fracture of Chaput's tubercle; PER 3 is characterised by a high fibular fracture (generally a simple fracture unlike in the PAB 3 fractures); PER 4 consists of rupture of the PITFL or a posterior malleolus fracture.

The final classification is the pronation–abduction (PAB) type ankle fracture (see separate station in Chapter 7). This has three stages, starting with the medial side (transverse avulsion type fracture of the medial malleolus or deep deltoid rupture), followed by an injury to the AITFL (or avulsion of Chaput's tubercle), with the final stage being characterised by a comminuted Weber C fracture of the fibula.

4. **In the context of a posterior malleolus fracture, when would you consider fixation?**

I would advocate fixation of a posterior malleolus fracture when it comprises >25% of the joint surface, or the talus is subluxed posteriorly. I would utilise two anterior to posterior screws inserted with a mini-open approach to avoid the multitude of tendons and neurovascular structures crossing the anterior ankle. If the fragment does not reduce closed, a posterolateral approach to the ankle would be employed to allow for open reduction, followed by application of a buttress plate.

FURTHER READING

Donken CC, Goorden AJ, Verhofstad MH, Edwards MJ. The outcome at 20 years of conservatively treated 'isolated' posterior malleolar fractures of the ankle: A case series. *J Bone Joint Surg Br.* 2011 Dec;93(12):1621–1625.

7

ANKLE FRACTURE

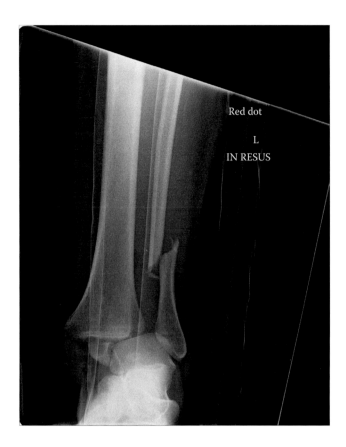

1. **Can you describe the radiograph?**

   This is an AP radiograph of the left ankle showing a fracture dislocation. There is an avulsion type fracture of the medial malleolus. There is an obvious diastasis at the distal tibiofibular syndesmosis and a spiral fracture of the fibula. This therefore represents a pronation–external rotation type injury.

2. **This is an isolated injury, with no neurovascular deficit. How would you manage this in the emergency department?**

   There is an obvious fracture dislocation of the ankle. To avoid swelling, which may preclude early surgical intervention in addition to protecting the cartilage and reducing patient discomfort preoperatively, I would advocate an emergent closed reduction under sedation in the emergency department by reversing the deformity. The leg will be placed in a below knee backslab, followed by check radiographs to confirm a satisfactory reduction of the talus. I would admit the patient to the ward for elevation +/– ice and discuss operative intervention with the patient.

3. What are the components to the syndesmosis of the ankle?

The syndesmosis of the ankle is the distal tibio–fibular joint. There are three components. Anteriorly, there is the anterior inferior tibio–fibular ligament (AITFL). Posteriorly, there is the posterior inferior tibio–fibular ligament (PITFL). Between these lies the interosseus ligament.

4. What form of treatment would you recommend?

This is a clearly unstable injury with an obvious syndesmosis injury. Assuming the patient has no contraindications to surgery, I would recommend operative intervention in order to provide the best chance of a relatively normal ankle in the future. It would be unlikely that a satisfactory position could be achieved in plaster, and even less likely that it would remain in that position. It would be important to counsel the patient in relation to the usual risks of surgery, in particular the risk of ongoing pain and stiffness owing to the severe nature of the injury.

The key to managing this injury is recognition of the syndesmosis injury. The syndesmosis requires particular care given the high rate of malreduction reported in the literature, with rates of over 50% reported (on postoperative CT scans). If the fibula can be reduced anatomically, the length and rotation of the fibula will be such that the syndesmosis is reduced and can be fixed in situ. My preferred method of fixation would be with a single small fragment (3.5 mm) screw, placed through three cortices, with no plan to remove the screw. The patient would be treated in a below knee cast, non-weight bearing for approximately 8 weeks.

In cases where there is dubiety over fibular reduction, for example, due to comminution, or in a Maisonneuve type injury, I would advocate an open approach to the syndesmosis to confirm the 'Mercedes Benz' sign, seen at the confluence of the tibia, fibula and talus. An alternative method would be to compare the image intensifier views of the injured side to the contralateral side intraoperatively. A true lateral of the talus on the contralateral side will show the appropriate relationship between the tibia and the fibula, and the AP view can determine the appropriate degree of tibiofibular overlap and fibular length. The latter can be assessed with talocrural angle and the 'dime sign'.

5. What factors determine your surgical outcome?

Outcome depends on anatomical reduction of the ankle mortise: 1 mm shift decreases contact by 42%. However, osteoarthritis – associated with instability or malreduction – is only symptomatic in approximately 10% of patients with radiographic changes.

Diabetic patients with poor diabetic control have a much higher rate of wound problems and deep infections.

One must also ensure that the syndesmosis is intact or fixed, otherwise this can lead to a severe and progressive valgus deformity.

FURTHER READING

Ganesh SP, Pietrobon R, Cecílio WA, Pan D et al. The impact of diabetes on patient outcomes after ankle fracture. *J Bone Joint Surg Am.* 2005 Aug;87(8):1712–1718.

Ramsey PL, Hamilton W. Changes in tibiotalar area of contact caused by lateral talar shift. *J Bone Joint Surg Am.* 1976 Apr;58(3):356–357.

8

INFECTED ANKLE

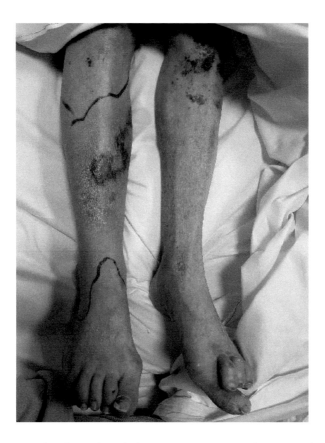

A 76-year-old non-insulin dependent diabetic returns to your clinic 3 weeks after ORIF of a right ankle fracture because he has been feeling unwell and has noticed redness and swelling extending beyond the plaster cast. This is a clinical photograph once the plaster cast has been removed.

1. **Describe this clinical picture.**

   This is a clinical photograph of both lower limbs. There is obvious pretibial erythema on the right side which has been marked out and this is suggestive of an extending cellulitis. The marked area includes the skin around the lateral malleolus. In addition, there are skin changes suggestive of chronic venous insufficiency affecting both legs with venous eczema and haemosiderin deposition bilaterally.

2. **How would you manage this patient in the outpatient clinic?**

   I would assess the patient fully looking particularly for signs of sepsis. I would take a history, asking specifically about any early wound problems and constitutional symptoms of infection such as fever, night sweats and loss of appetite. I would ask the nurses to perform a full set of observations. I would remove any remaining dressings and would clean and examine the wound before applying a clean saline dressing. I would assess the vascularity of the foot using a handheld Doppler for pedal pulses. I would obtain radiographs of the ankle and would take blood samples for full blood count, inflammatory markers (CRP and ESR) and blood cultures. I would then admit the patient.

3. **What would be your definitive management for this patient?**

This fracture will not yet have united and there is now obvious evidence of infection. I would attempt to suppress the infection in the first instance using intravenous antibiotics. The success of this strategy would be dependent upon identifying the responsible bacteria and targeting them with appropriate antibiotics. If the wound has only minimal ooze or none then I would send a wound swab for microbiology examination and treat appropriately. If there is more significant drainage, any suggestion of a collection or if the patient fails to respond to initial targeted therapy then I would take the patient to the operating theatre, wash out and debride the wound, apply a negative pressure dressing and send samples for microbiology analysis. I would hope that this would allow the fracture to unite after which I could arrange to remove the metalwork. Repeat wound examination and renewal of the dressing will be required after 48 hours. Premature removal of the metalwork may result in an infected non-union, a much more difficult problem to treat. Nevertheless, if the infection cannot be suppressed with antibiotics, it may still be necessary to remove the metalwork.

As part of the more general management of the patient, his diabetic control should be optimised and I would recruit the assistance of the diabetic nurse specialist and medical team. Attention to footwear, ulcers and pressure areas as well as the local vascularity of the foot are also important. A neurological assessment and pedal pulses should be examined for and recorded preoperatively. Doppler assessment should be used where pulses cannot be confidently identified.

FURTHER READING

Ovaska MT, Mäkinen TJ, Madanat R, Vahlberg T, Hirvensalo E, Lindahl J. Predictors of poor outcomes following deep infection after internal fixation of ankle fractures. *Injury*. 2013 Jul;44(7):1002–1006.

Wukich DK, Lowery NJ, McMillen RL, Frykberg RG. Postoperative infection rates in foot and ankle surgery: A comparison of patients with and without diabetes mellitus. *J Bone Joint Surg Am*. 2010 Feb;92(2):287–295.

9

PILON FRACTURE

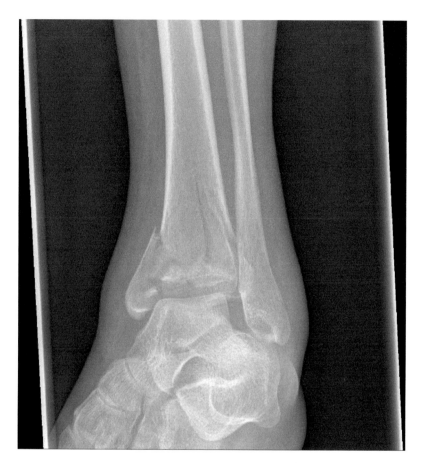

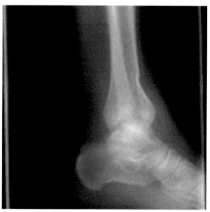

1. Describe the radiographs pictured above.

These are AP and lateral radiographs showing a comminuted and displaced pilon fracture. There is articular impaction and comminution, as well as metaphyseal comminution, as is typical with most pilon fractures.

2. What is the typical mechanism of injury?

The mechanism of injury is axial load. They are usually sustained as a result of a high-energy injury, commonly after a fall from height or a motor vehicle accident.

3. How would you manage this injury initially?

This is a high-energy injury with the potential for other life- or limb-threatening injuries. I would manage this patient in the emergency department as per ATLS guidelines with concurrent assessment and treatment using an ABCDE approach. The limb itself must be carefully inspected and assessed for the degree of soft tissue injury as this will be the deciding factor in how to manage the fracture initially.

After sufficient analgesia, I would perform a circumferential examination of the limb, looking for any evidence of open injury and documenting the degree of skin damage, contusion or fracture blistering. A thorough neurovascular examination should be performed. This would include palpation of the posterior tibial artery and dorsalis pedis artery, as well as an examination of the capillary refill to ensure an intact vascular supply, followed by examination of the five nerves to cross the ankle joint: superficial and deep peroneal nerves; tibial nerve (which branches into the medial and lateral plantar nerves to supply the sole); sural nerve and the saphenous nerve.

Any skin tenting or impending breaches would be managed emergently with a closed reduction under sedation in the emergency department. Compartment syndrome is less common in pilon fractures than tibial shaft fractures but would require a high index of suspicion to ensure early recognition.

Assuming that this is an isolated injury, a closed reduction would be performed prior to placing the patient into a plaster of Paris backslab for immobilisation, pain relief and limb/fracture alignment. The hindfoot should be aligned with the tibia and any rotational deformity corrected.

4. Would you want any further investigations prior to determining your treatment of choice?

A CT scan would allow for better visualisation of the fracture configuration, particularly the intra-articular component, and is vital for preoperative planning. If these are greatly displaced, a CT scan following spanning external fixation is generally more useful.

5. How can one classify such injuries?

There is no commonly accepted classification for intra-articular fractures of the distal tibia. Two classification systems that can be applied include the AO classification or the Ruedi and Allgower classification.

The former system allocates 4-3 to the distal tibia (four for tibia and three for the distal portion). 43A fractures are extra-articular and therefore not true pilon fractures as the plafond is unaffected. 43B refers to partial articular fractures and 43C refers to complete articular fractures. C type fractures are further subdivided into C1 (simple articular), C2 (simple articular, complex metaphyseal) and C3 (complex articular, complex metaphyseal).

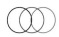

The latter classification system is divided into types I, II or III. Type I is an undisplaced pilon fracture, type II is a fracture with significant joint incongruity but without comminution, and type III is a comminuted intra-articular fracture.

6. What are the common intra-articular fragments associated with a pilon fracture?
These are

I – Anterolateral fragment (Chaput fragment). This is the attachment of the anterior inferior tibiofibular ligament

II – Posterolateral fragment (Volkmann fragment). This is the attachment of the posterior inferior tibiofibular ligament

III – Medial malleolus. This is the attachment of the deltoid ligament

IV – Die punch fragment. This is the central articular fragment which lacks soft tissue attachment and therefore cannot be reduced by ligamentotaxis. It can prevent reduction and must be addressed by direct visualisation. These fragments vary in size and number depending on the degree of comminution.

7. How would you manage this after an initial closed reduction in the emergency department, assuming it's a closed and neurovascularly intact injury?
The treatment of pilon fractures is complex and many different treatment options are described, both for initial management and definitive management.

If the patient is fit for surgical management and has a displaced fracture, I would discuss operative treatment with the patient. However, there is controversy regarding the timing of surgery for these complex, high-energy, intra-articular injuries. One must decide between a 'span and scan' method of treatment or early ORIF. In the former, a spanning external fixator is applied to the affected limb prior to obtaining a CT scan and planning for conversion to ORIF once swelling has subsided, the soft tissue envelope is healthy, and there is no evidence of pin site infection.

For the 'span and scan' approach, I would insert two tibial shaft half pins (away from the zone of injury). I would incise the skin then spread the soft tissues bluntly down to bone. I would use a sharp drill bit with a sleeve and irrigate whilst predrilling the cortex to avoid heat damage, before finally inserting the appropriate pin using a sleeve. This would be followed by the calcaneal transfixion pin into the calcaneal tuberosity, from medial to lateral, to protect the NV structures behind the medial malleolus. To prevent an equinus deformity of the ankle, a single 4 mm pin can be inserted into the base of the first metatarsal. I would connect these pins using clamps and rods to reduce the fracture and maintain that ankle at 90 degrees.

Ultimately, the decision between early ORIF and 'span-and-scan' depends on a multitude of factors, the most important of which are the state of the soft tissues, the mechanism of injury, the patient's physiological age and co-morbidities, and the availability of expertise to treat this complex injury.

The principles of the definitive surgery are to restore anatomical reduction of the articular surface, reconnect the articular surface to the metaphysis, and then the metaphysis to the diaphysis, whilst protecting the soft tissue envelope. ORIF as both initial and definitive management requires an honest assessment of the state of the soft tissues.

My favoured approach for ORIF of a pilon fracture is the anteromedial approach. It is the workhorse approach to the ankle as it's extensile and can be used for future surgery such as potential ankle fusion or ankle arthroplasty.

In some cases, a posterolateral approach to the tibia is required initially where there is a displaced posterior malleolus fragment. The patient is placed prone and the internervous plane between FHL (tibial nerve) and the peroneal tendons (superficial peroneal nerve) is utilised to expose, reduce and buttress the fragment. The posterior malleolus fragment can then be used as the keystone for reconstruction through an anteromedial approach. If required, the fibula may be reduced and fixed through this same incision.

8. Can you describe the anterior approach to the ankle and how you would reduce and fix the fracture?

The patient is placed supine with a pneumatic thigh tourniquet. An incision is placed just medial to the tibialis anterior, starting approximately 10 cm proximal to the ankle joint and extending over the ankle joint towards the second ray. The extensor retinaculum is incised and the tibialis anterior tendon sheath is kept intact to minimise wound problems. The plane between EHL (medially) and EDL (laterally) is identified. The NV bundle (anterior tibial artery and deep peroneal nerve) lies between these two tendons just proximal to the ankle and is behind EHL at the level of the ankle joint. EHL and the NV bundle are retracted medially and EDL is retracted laterally. The ankle joint capsule is incised in line with the incision and the full width of the ankle joint can be exposed by subperiosteal dissection.

The fracture is opened to expose the die punch fragment which must be reduced and held to the posterior malleolus to prevent it from blocking reduction of the main fragments. The remaining fragments are provisionally fixed to the posterior malleolus with K-wires and clamps, before fixing these definitively with a site-specific locking plate. My preference is for an anterolateral plate, as opposed to an anteromedial plate over which there would be little soft tissue coverage.

Where there is difficulty reducing the fracture fragments, application of a distractor can help with visualisation of the articular surface and may also align several of the major articular fragments. One Schanz pin is placed into the talus and the other into the tibia.

9. What other options exist for definitive management of pilon fractures?

An external fixator or circular frame may be used. However, there is a higher rate of mal-union associated with external fixator use and the inability to reduce the die punch fragment leads to less anatomical reconstruction of the articular surface. However, clinical trials have failed to show conclusive superiority of ORIF or external fixation.

10. How would you manage a fibular fracture associated with a pilon fracture?

Fibular fractures associated with pilon-type injuries to the distal tibia can be managed in a number of ways. They can be managed conservatively, reduced and fixed with a view to helping re-establish lateral column length or the fibula can be taken as bone graft used to augment external fixation.

A retrospective case control study from a level-one trauma centre in the United States could find no significant difference in outcomes among three groups: Fibular fixation, no fibular fixation, no fibular fracture. The only difference was that the group who underwent fibular fixation had a statistically higher rate of metalwork removal.

11. What are the complications of this injury when managed operatively?

Starting with early complications, these would include wound dehiscence and infection, particularly in open fractures or where the state of the soft tissue envelope is not respected preoperatively. Compartment syndrome, although rare in this type of injury, may complicate the early pre- or postoperative period.

Late complications secondary OA, delayed union, mal-union (more common with external fixation than ORIF) and non-union. Indolent infection can present as delayed or non-union and may cause osteomyelitis associated with infected metalwork.

FURTHER READING

Kurlyo JC, Datta N, Iskander KN, Tornetta P III. Does the fibular need to be fixed in complex pilon fractures? *J Orthop Trauma*. 2015 Sep;29(9):424–427.

MIDSHAFT DIAPHYSEAL TIBIA FRACTURE

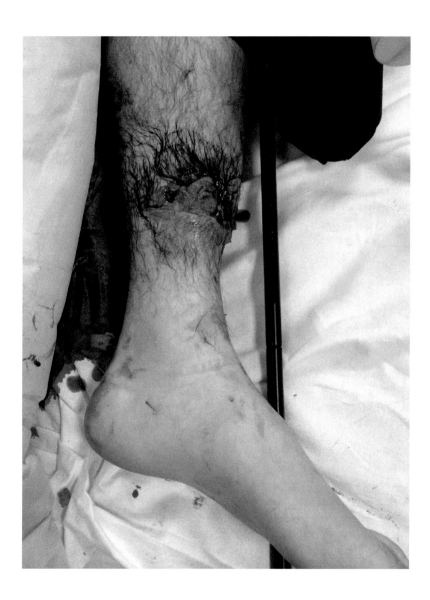

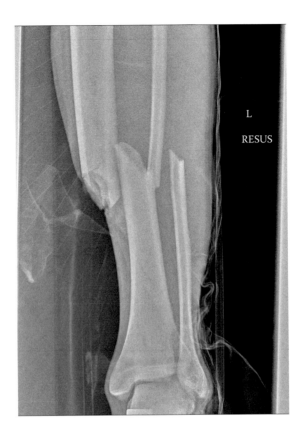

A 40-year-old woman is struck by a motorcycle while crossing the road. She is brought to the emergency department shortly after 10 p.m. These are her radiographs and clinical photographs of her leg.

1. **Describe the photographs and x-rays.**
   The clinical photographs show the left leg, which is swollen and deformed. There is a wound over the anteromedial aspect of the middle third of the leg. The radiograph show a displaced and comminuted fracture of the midshaft of the tibia. The clinical photograph and radiograph clearly indicate an open fracture.

2. **Describe your initial investigation and management.**
   This is a high-energy injury and the patient should be treated along established ATLS principles. With respect to this specific injury I would take a careful history from the patient and examine the limb looking to confirm the state of the soft tissues, any gross contamination which I would remove, additional wounds or soft tissue injury, the neurovascular status of the limb and any features suggestive of compartment syndrome. I would look closely for any fracture or instability affecting the femur, patella, hip or adjacent joints.

   Guidelines for the management of severe lower limb injuries have been formalised by the BOA/BAPRAS and are summarised in BOAST 4. I would take a clinical photograph of the limb before dressing the wound with saline-soaked gauze and splinting the limb in an above knee backslab. I would administer intravenous cefuroxime (1.5 g) and tetanus toxoid. I would request periodic assessments for pain, evidence of compartment syndrome and the neurovascular status of the limb. I would perform a complete secondary survey.

This patient will require surgery. I would prepare them for surgical wound debridement and fracture stabilisation as a joint case with orthopaedic and plastic surgery input on the routine trauma list the following day.

3. How would you manage this injury and patient definitively?

Having confirmed that this is an isolated injury, I would obtain consent from the patient for wound debridement and surgical stabilisation. This would be performed with my plastic surgery colleagues the next day during working hours unless there was a limb-threatening injury such as a vascular injury needing repair or developing compartment syndrome when emergent surgery would be necessary. Regular intravenous cefuroxime (750 mg) is given eight hourly until the debridement is performed. The debridement includes extension of the wound as required in order to allow a formal assessment of the soft and bony tissues in theatre where contaminated or devitalised tissue is removed and I would wash the wound out with at least 6 litres of warmed saline. Loose bony fragments are assessed by the 'tug test' to see if they have any appreciable soft tissue attachments and by implication, a blood supply to suggest that they remain viable.

Following the debridement, the soft tissue envelope and bony stability are reassessed. Options for surgical stabilisation would include a temporary external fixator, reamed intramedullary nailing or Ilizarov or Taylor Spatial Frame. Where the wound can be safely closed or covered at the index procedure, my preference would be to treat this with an intramedullary nail. Antibiotics are continued until definitive wound closure or for 72 hours, whichever occurs soonest, and close observation is required for any signs of compartment syndrome.

FURTHER READING

British Association of Plastic, Reconstructive and Aesthetic Surgeons (BAPRAS). Management of severe open lower limb fractures. Accessed from https://www.boa.ac.uk/wp-content/uploads/2014/05/BOAST-4-The-Management-of-Sever-Open-Lower-Limb-Fractures.pdf.

British Association of Plastic, Reconstructive and Aesthetic Surgeons (BAPRAS). Open fractures of the lower limb. Accessed from http://www.bapras.org.uk/professionals/clinical-guidance/open-fractures-of-the-lower-limb.

Court-Brown CM, Will E, Christie J, McQueen MM. Reamed or unreamed nailing for closed tibial fractures. A prospective study in Tscherne C1 fractures. *J Bone Joint Surg Br.* 1996 Jul;78(4):580–583.

Naique SB, Pearse M, Nanchahal J. Management of severe open tibial fractures: The need for combined orthopaedic and plastic surgical treatment in specialist centres. *J Bone Joint Surg Br.* 2006 Mar;88(3):351–357.

Schemitsch EH, Bhandari M, Guyatt G, Sanders DW, Swiontkowski M, Tornetta P III, Walter SD, Zdero R, Goslings JC, Teague D, Jeray K, McKee MD. Study to Prospectively Evaluate Reamed Intramedullary Nails in Patients with Tibial Fractures (SPRINT) Investigators. Prognostic factors for predicting outcomes after intramedullary nailing of the tibia. *J Bone Joint Surg Am.* 2012 Oct 3;94(19):1786–1793. doi: 10.2106/JBJS.J.01418.

11

COMPARTMENT SYNDROME

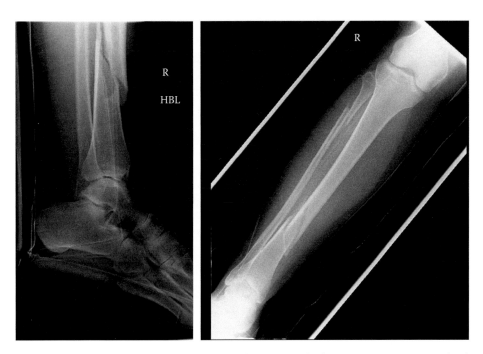

You are the on-call orthopaedic registrar and you are asked to see a young man who has been brought to the emergency department after a direct collision with another player on the football pitch.

1. **This is his radiograph, which shows his only injury. Can you tell me what is going on here and how you would manage this in the first instance?**
   This is an AP and lateral radiograph of a right tibia showing a displaced mid-diaphyseal tibial fracture. I would make a full clinical assessment taking a history and performing a full examination with particular reference to any open wounds. I would also perform and record a neurovascular examination and specifically look to exclude compartment syndrome. If this was all satisfactory, I would ensure that the patient had adequate analgesia before splinting them in an above knee backslab. I would admit them to the ward area. I would plan to manage this fracture with intramedullary nailing and I would mark and consent the patient for this to be performed on the next routine trauma list.

2. **You are called to reassess the patient on the ward just after 1 a.m. because he has been complaining of pain and is requiring considerable amounts of opioid analgesia. What do you think might be going on and how would you proceed?**
   This presentation is typical of compartment syndrome, which can be associated with tibial fractures. I would reassess the patient. The predominant presenting feature of compartment syndrome is pain out of proportion to that which would be expected from the injury alone. Paresthesiae, pallor, paralysis and pulselessness may

all be additional late signs. Compartment syndrome is a clinical diagnosis but if there is doubt as to the diagnosis, I might consider compartment pressure monitoring. Increased opioid consumption is a warning sign. Pain is exacerbated by passive stretch of the muscles in the affected compartment, in this case, the extensor hallucis longus, toe extensors and tibialis anterior. Having confirmed the diagnosis clinically I would consent and mark the patient to undergo emergent fasciotomies and intramedullary nailing of the fracture at the same sitting.

3. **Can you tell me how you would perform your fasciotomies and where you would place your incisions?**
   I would perform a two-incision four-compartment fasciotomy. In an appropriately marked and consented patient, I would position the patient on a radiolucent table suitable for subsequent freehand intramedullary nailing. I would initially place a sandbag under the ipsilateral hip to roll the leg into slight internal rotation and I would make my lateral incision first.
   The lateral skin incision is placed halfway between the tibial crest and the subcutaneous surface of the fibula so that is anterior to the fibula and it is an extensile incision along the length of the leg. I would 'spread' through fat onto the fascial layer, being careful not to injure the superficial peroneal nerve, although if it is not apparent I will not specifically look for it or dissect it out. I would expect to find it 5–10 cm proximal to the lateral malleolus. I feel for the lateral intermuscular septum to identify the demarcation between the anterior and lateral compartments and then retract the skin flaps to incise the fascial layer longitudinally over each compartment. I would then inspect and palpate to ensure there are no taut bands of fascia remaining. The diagnosis is often confirmed at the time of surgery by a tight compartment, bulging muscle or sometimes apparent muscle necrosis. I would assess the muscle compartments for colour, consistency, capacity to bleed and contractility.
   I would then move to the medial side and I would pack the lateral wounds with saline-soaked swabs and ask for the sandbag to be removed. I would site my medial skin incision 1 cm posterior to the medial border of the tibia aiming to protect perforating vessels and to come anterior to the posterior tibial artery. Again, this is an extensile incision, along the length of the leg, and I would aim to leave an adequate skin bridge of at least 7 cm between incisions. I would dissect down to the fascial layer and divide this in the line of the skin incision to decompress the superficial posterior compartment. I would then retract or bluntly dissect the superficial compartment muscles off the deep compartment to expose the fascia overlying the deep compartment and I would incise this as well, releasing the muscle completely.
   Importantly, the wounds are not closed and after the tibial fracture has been treated with nailing, the wounds are dressed with a negative pressure dressing. The patient is brought back to the operating theatre for wound inspection, debridement if required and possible wound closure at 48 hours as a planned procedure with plastic surgeons in attendance. If early closure is not possible at the first inspection, I would plan to undertake a second inspection at a further 48 hours with a plastic surgeon and be prepared to proceed with split skin grafting if necessary. The patient remains on intravenous antibiotics until the wounds are closed.

4. **Assuming the diagnosis was delayed for several days after tibial nailing in the same patient, how would you manage this?**
   This is a difficult decision. There is very little evidence to guide the management of a delayed diagnosis of compartment syndrome. In this situation, the aim is to

minimise morbidity and to salvage limb function. If it is apparent that there is established complete muscle necrosis then there is little benefit in performing fasciotomies which may expose the patient to wound problems. If the degree of muscle necrosis is not felt to be so severe then fasciotomies may be undertaken to prevent further muscle loss and to allow debridement of necrotic tissue. Severe systemic upset, rhabdomyolysis and even renal failure may be indications for life-saving surgery where fasciotomies, debridement or even amputation may be required.

FURTHER READING

McQueen MM, Duckworth AD, Aitken SA, Sharma RA, Court-Brown CM. Predictors of compartment syndrome after tibial fracture. *J Orthop Trauma*. 2015 Oct;29(10):451–455.

Whitesides TE, Haney TC, Morimoto K, Harada H. Tissue pressure measurements as a determinant for the need of fasciotomy. *Clin Orthop Relat Res*. 1975 Nov–Dec;(113):43–51.

White TO, Howell GE, Will EM, Court-Brown CM, McQueen MM. Elevated intramuscular compartment pressures do not influence outcome after tibial fracture. *J Trauma*. 2003 Dec;55(6):1133–1138.

12

TIBIAL DIAPHYSEAL FRACTURE (PROXIMAL)

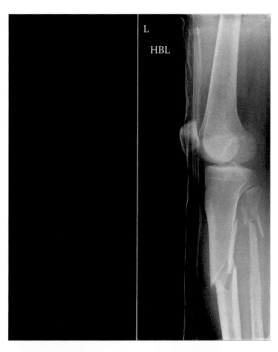

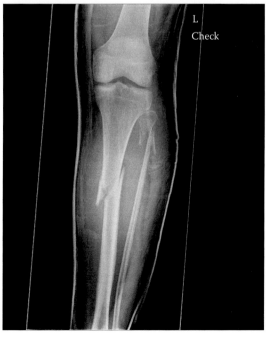

1. **Can you describe the radiographs?**

   These are AP and lateral radiographs of the left tibia and fibula showing a proximal tibial diaphyseal fracture. The fracture is in valgus and procurvatum (apex anterior).

2. **What is responsible for the deformities seen here?**

   The procurvatum is due to the unopposed pull of the patellar tendon, whereas the valgus deformity is due to the pull of the pes anserinus attached to the proximal fragment, and the bulky anterior compartment musculature preventing the fracture from displacing into a varus configuration.

3. **If you were to treat this fracture with an IM nail, what techniques could you use to counteract these deformities?**

   There are several techniques one could utilise to prevent this valgus and procurvatum deformity. Since the nail is not in contact with the cortical bone at the level of the fracture, the fragment can displace until the posterior or lateral cortex lies in contact with the nail:

   a. Poller* blocking screws: These are bicortical screws inserted before reaming and nailing. Alternatives include thick K-wires or 3/16-inch smooth Steinmann Pins. The screw/wire/pin blocks the incorrect path of the nail and channels the nail along the correct path preventing a mal-union. In the case of the fracture pictured above, a poller screw placed posteriorly will prevent the procurvatum deformity and a lateral screw will prevent the valgus deformity.

   b. Unicortical plate: A mini-open approach can be utilised to reduce the fracture and maintain fixation using a small fragment dynamic compression plate with unicortical fixation.

   c. Lateral starting point: A lateral parapatellar approach and lateral proximal starting point will allow the nail to abut the lateral cortex of the proximal fragment and prevent a valgus deformity.

   d. Semi-extended nailing: Nailing with the knee in flexion can exaggerate any procurvatum deformity. Most companies can now supply instrumentation to allow for nailing of tibial fractures in a semi-extended position, preventing fracture malalignment.

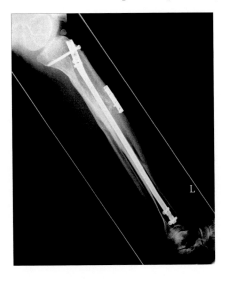

---

* *Poller* is German for bollard.

13

MANGLED EXTREMITY

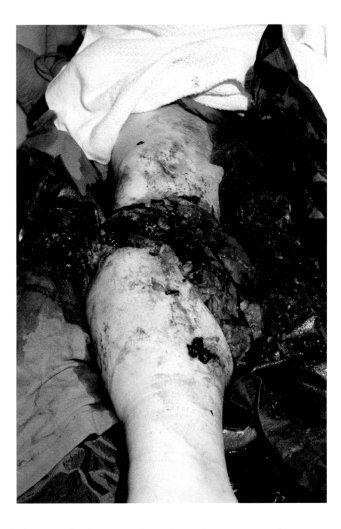

This is a clinical photograph of a patient brought to the emergency department after being hit by a car that crushed and pinned his leg to a wall.

1. **Describe this clinical picture.**

   This is a clinical photograph of a patient with an obviously mangled and deformed leg. The wounds are ragged and the soft tissues appear dusky. There is obvious bone and soft tissue loss. It is not possible to tell from this photograph if this is an isolated injury.

2. **Assuming that this is an isolated injury, how would you manage this patient in the emergency department?**

   This patient would be treated along ATLS principles with concurrent resuscitation to treat life- and limb-threatening injuries and to address any catastrophic haemorrhage early. I would address active haemorrhage from the wound with limb elevation and direct pressure and the use of a tourniquet if required. I would treat the patient with intravenous fluid and blood resuscitation as required and activate our major haemorrhage protocol if clinically indicated based on the patient's initial state, response to resuscitation and mechanism of injury triggers as per our local major haemorrhage policy. I would administer intravenous antibiotics, tetanus toxoid and analgesia. A clinical photograph should be taken before gross contamination is removed and saline swab dressings and a bandage are applied. Radiographs to confirm the bony injury and to help identify any proximal foreign body contamination should be taken. I would carefully assess and record the neurovascular status and include an assessment of pulses with Doppler ultrasound.

I would look closely for any suggestion of compartment syndrome, and an early senior surgical opinion is required as to whether limb salvage or early amputation for trauma is required. In any case, I would plan to take this patient to the operating theatre to perform a wound debridement. I would plan to provide temporary stability using an external fixator or plaster of Paris, but I would also consent the patient for amputation of the limb.

3. How would you decide between limb salvage and primary amputation?

There are a number of scoring systems to guide this decision. The Mangled Extremity Scoring System (MESS) is the most widely known but has largely fallen from favour. Loss of plantar sensation has also been used as a predictor of a poor outcome for limb salvage, as indicative of injury to the posterior tibial nerve, but this is also no longer used since the LEAP study demonstrated that at 2 years almost 50% of patients regained some plantar sensation.

The agreement of two experienced surgeons as to the need for amputation should be sought. In general, absolute indications for amputation are taken to include a contaminated traumatic amputation, a mangled extremity in a shocked and severely injured patient, and a crushed extremity with arterial injury and a warm ischemia time of greater than 6 hours. Relative indications include severe bone or soft-tissue loss, an anatomic transection of the tibial nerve, an open tibial fracture with serious associated polytrauma or a severe ipsilateral foot injury, or a prolonged predicted course to obtain soft-tissue coverage and tibial reconstruction. Despite this, the LEAP study suggests that the outcomes for both limb salvage and primary amputation are poor and that there is a high complication and re-operation rate. Where there is doubt about the state of limb perfusion, a CT angiogram can be helpful, but this should not introduce unnecessary delay in moving to the operating theatre to undertake debridement, restore limb perfusion if required and stabilisation.

4. At what level would you plan to undertake this amputation and what are the principles that would guide your surgery?

Current guidance from the BOA and BAPRAS is that open tibial fractures should be operated on within 24 hours with a combined 'orthoplastic' approach. Surgery should be undertaken more urgently if there is gross contamination or an arterial injury requiring repair. The level of amputation should be guided by the soft tissue injury and the level at which adequate soft tissue coverage can be obtained. Preservation of length improves energy expenditure during rehabilitation for the patient but should not compromise the adequacy of the debridement. In a clean wound, it would be usual to perform a definitive procedure at the time, fashioning flaps at the index surgery. For this injury, it may be possible to undertake a below knee amputation. For crush, blast or grossly contaminated injuries, the evidence suggests that flaps should not be fashioned at the index procedure and at least one further debridement should be undertaken to reduce the risks of subsequent infection, retained contamination or flap failure.

FURTHER READING

BOA. 2009. Standards for the management of open fractures of the lower limb. BAPRAS 1–24. Accessed from http://www.boa.ac.uk/site/showpublications.aspx?id=59.

Bosse MJ, McCarthy ML, Jones AL et al. The insensate foot following severe lower extremity trauma: An indication for amputation? *J Bone Joint Surg.* 2005;87-A:2601–2608.

Gustilo RB, Mendoza RM, Williams DN. Problems in the management of type III (severe) open fractures: A new classification of type III open fractures. *J Trauma.* 1984;24:742–746.

Tintle SM, Keeling JJ, Shawen SB, Forsberg JA, Potter BK. Traumatic and trauma-related amputations: Part I: General principles and lower-extremity amputations. *J Bone Joint Surg Am.* 2010 Dec 1;92(17):2852–2868. Review.

14

TIBIAL PLATEAU FRACTURE

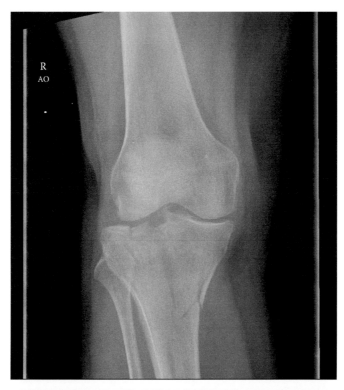

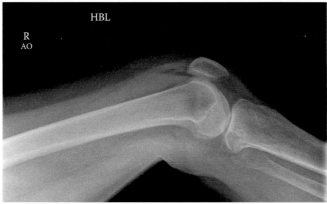

These are the radiographs for a patient involved in a high-energy road traffic accident.

1. **Describe the appearance in these radiographs.**
   These are AP and lateral radiographs of the right knee. There is an obvious fracture of the tibial plateau affecting both the medial and lateral compartments.

2. How would you manage and investigate this patient initially?

This represents a high-energy injury and this patient would be received and treated in the emergency department along ATLS principles.

With respect to this specific injury I would ensure that the patient is given adequate analgesia. I would perform a full circumferential examination of the limb paying attention to the state of the soft tissues to identify the degree of soft tissue swelling, any open wounds, blistering or degloving. I would make an assessment of the neurovascular status.

Assuming this is a closed injury without neurovascular deficit, I would then splint the limb using plaster of Paris in an above knee backslab. I would be careful to look for associated injuries to the knee, ankle and foot. It may be difficult to assess for ligamentous injuries of the knee at this time, but I would remain suspicious.

I suspect that this patient may require operative treatment and a CT scan of the knee would help with preoperative planning. I would also make an assessment for and request continued clinical assessments of the potential for development of compartment syndrome.

3. What are the treatment options for this patient?

This is a highly comminuted and displaced fracture with disruption of a weight bearing joint. Non-operative treatment is an option depending on the overall condition of the patient but in a fit and healthy patient I would recommend operative fixation should the condition of the patient and the soft tissues permit this.

I would expect that this fracture pattern would be amenable to fixation with locked peri articular plates but this would need to be confirmed by the CT scan. Should this not be the case, Ilizarov or Taylor Spatial Frame fixation may be alternatives. There is also some evidence for primary arthroplasty as a treatment for elderly patients with tibial plateau fractures and pre-existing knee arthritis.

4. Can you describe your patient positioning and surgical approach for operative fixation?

In an appropriately marked and consented patient under general anaesthesia, I would request that intravenous antibiotics are administered before a thigh tourniquet is applied and inflated. I would position the patient supine on an operating table that is broken so that the knees are flexed to 90 degrees. A small sterile or wrapped bolster under the knee would assist in obtaining unobstructed lateral radiographs.

I would make a straight midline skin incision passing posteriorly and laterally just proximal to the joint line in a gentle hockey stick curvilinear fashion. This allows the origin of the muscles in the anterior compartment to be released. The approach raises thick flaps down to the joint capsule. The joint capsule is opened through a sub-meniscal arthrotomy. The meniscus is then lifted out of the field of view using a stay stitch to allow the articular surface to be visualised. Alternatively, the anterior horn of the meniscus may be divided, tagged and subsequently repaired to allow access.

This approach allows good access to lateral plateau fractures. Depressed articular portions of the plateau can be reduced by raising the joint through a metaphyseal window using a punch.

I would use a separate posteromedial incision to allow access and reduction of the medial plateau fracture. I would fix this using an additional plate. The skin incision for this approach is based on a line along the posteromedial border of the tibia extending just proximal to the joint line. This leaves a suitable skin bridge. The tendons of the pes anserinus are retracted out of the way distally although the semi-membranosus may need to be divided, tagged and subsequently repaired. The plane anterior to the medial head of gastrocnemius is identified and developed. Remaining in this plane protects the popliteal vessels allowing me to safely dissect down to the joint capsule and open the joint. On the occasions when the medial plateau fracture is undisplaced, this can often be satisfactorily fixed from the lateral side using a locking plate unless there is a large posteromedial fragment which would typically have a large portion of joint surface associated with it.

5. **What are the potential complications of operative treatment?**
These include wound problems or breakdown, neurovascular injury, bleeding, infection, deep venous thrombosis and pulmonary embolism. Pin tract infection is associated with external fixation. In addition, joint stiffness, painful or prominent metalwork, secondary surgery or removal of metalwork, mal-union and post-traumatic arthritis may all occur.

6. **What weight bearing status or restrictions would you recommend?**
I would protect the fixation with a period of 6 weeks non-weight bearing in a hinged knee brace set between 0 and 90 degrees of flexion in order to maintain range of movement followed by a gradual increase in weight bearing and range of movement with physiotherapy supervision. More comminuted fracture types or where the fixation is tenuous may require a longer period of protection.

FURTHER READING

Egol KA, Su E, Tejwani NC, Sims SH, Kummer FJ, Koval KJ. Treatment of complex tibial plateau fractures using the less invasive stabilization system plate: Clinical experience and a laboratory comparison with double plating. *J Trauma.* 2004 Aug;57(2):340–346.

Gosling T, Schandelmaier P, Muller M, Hankemeier S, Wagner M, Krettek C. Single lateral locked screw plating of bicondylar tibial plateau fractures. *Clin Orthop Relat Res.* 2005 Oct;439:207–214.

Higgins TF, Kemper D, Klatt J. Incidence and morphology of the posteromedial fragment in bicondylar tibial plateau fractures. *J Orthop Trauma.* 2009 Jan;23(1):45–51. doi: 10.1097/BOT.0b013e31818f8dc1.

15
KNEE DISLOCATION

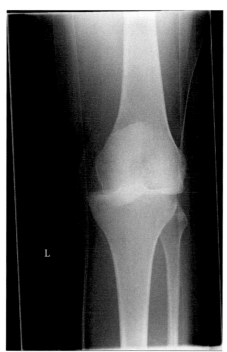

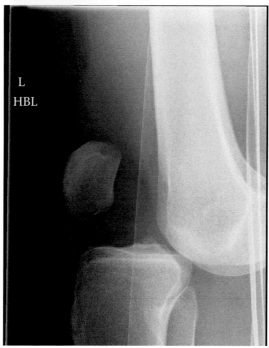

1. **Can you describe the radiographs and tell me what your immediate concerns would be?**

   These are AP and lateral radiographs of a left knee showing an anterior knee dislocation. My immediate concern for this patient would be that this injury may be part of a high-energy injury. I would manage them in line with ATLS guidelines in order to ensure that all life- and limb-threatening injuries are identified and prioritised. My immediate concern for the affected limb would be the neurovascular status. An arterial injury, although less common than a nerve injury, may require surgical intervention with disastrous complications (including amputation) if missed. Approximately 25% have a common peroneal nerve injury.

2. **How would you assess and manage this patient initially?**

   As already mentioned, if this is a high-energy injury, I would manage the patient according to ATLS guidelines. Prior to reduction, I would assess and document the neurovascular status of the limb and assess for a 'dimple' sign, which is indicative of an irreducible reduction; the medial femoral condyle has buttonholed through the medial capsule. Delayed reduction risks skin necrosis. I would then attempt closed reduction under sedation as an emergency before repeating my neurovascular assessment and confirming a satisfactory reduction with repeat radiographs.

   There is no universally agreed management protocol for suspected arterial injuries. Signs of an arterial injury include reduced pulse volume or frank absence of pulses, cool toes with a slow capillary refill, an expanding haematoma around the knee, or an ankle-brachial pressure index (ABPI) <0.9, all of which warrant an urgent vascular review. Patients with these findings require urgent vascular surgical advice which may include angiography. Numerous case series have shown angiography to be superfluous in the context of an entirely normal clinical examination as above.

   Even in the presence of a normal vascular examination, the patient will require serial examinations on the ward as an intimal injury may progress to critical ischaemia.

3. **How would you proceed if this patient had a confirmed arterial injury?**

   Patients who sustain vascular injuries associated with a knee dislocation require urgent transfer to a trauma hospital and urgent revascularisation. I would apply a spanning external fixator to maintain a secure reduction prior to the vascular surgeons performing a vascular repair. The vascular surgeons may wish to perform a vascular shunt prior to application of the external fixator.

4. **Why is the popliteal artery at particular risk of injury with knee dislocations?**

   The popliteal artery is strongly tethered in the region of the popliteal fossa, proximally by the fibrous tunnel at the adductor hiatus, and distally at the fibrous tunnel at the soleus arch.

5. **How are knee dislocations classified?**

   These injuries can be classified as above (where the dislocation is described in the context of the direction of tibial movement in relation to the femur) or using the knee dislocation (KD) classification proposed by Schenck:

   > KD I – Multiligamentous knee injury with only one cruciate ligament involved
   >
   > KD II – Both cruciates ruptured, but no other ligamentous injury (rare)

KD III – Both cruciates ruptured, plus either the medial collateral ligament (MCL) or lateral collateral ligament (LCL) (three ligaments injured)

KD IV – Both cruciates and both collateral ligaments ruptured (four ligaments injured)

KD V – Multiligamentous injury with periarticular fracture

6. **How would you investigate and manage this definitively?**

I would arrange for this patient to have a preoperative MRI in order to confirm the nature of the ligamentous injury as well as rule out associated meniscal or osteochondral pathology. I would arrange a CT scan if there was suspicion of fracture on the plain radiographs.

Non-operative management results in a high incidence of recurrent instability, arthrofibrosis and pain, with low outcome scores. In the absence of any contraindications, I would advise repair/reconstruction of the ligamentous injuries performed by a soft tissue knee surgeon with experience in this area.

The most recent evidence is in the form of the largest case series to date with a 10-year follow-up: The group performed early surgical intervention in 40 patients and followed them up to determine outcomes. The algorithm used in this study required reconstruction of the posterolateral corner by means of an open approach followed by an arthroscopically assisted reconstruction of the ACL and PCL. There is an increased risk of compartment syndrome resulting from the high-energy nature of injury together with prolonged surgery and the potential for extravasation of fluid during the arthroscopically assisted reconstruction of the cruciate ligaments. The skin wounds remained open during the arthroscopy to allow controlled drainage of the saline and a tourniquet break for reperfusion was used as required.

7. **If the patient had a common peroneal nerve injury at the time of presentation, how would you manage this and what would you tell the patient?**

Unfortunately, these injuries have a poor prognosis. Managed expectantly, one-third will return to normal, one-third will undergo partial recovery, and one-third will display no recovery. I would explain this to the patient, as well as future management options, which may include nerve grafting, functional orthoses or tendon transfers.

FURTHER READING

Khakha RS, Day AC, Gibbs J, Allen S et al. Acute surgical management of traumatic knee dislocations – Average follow-up of 10 years. *Knee*. 2016 Mar;23(2):267–275.

Medina O, Arom GA, Yeranosian MG, Petrigliano FA et al. Vascular and nerve injury after knee dislocation: A systematic review. *Clin Orthop Relat Res*. 2014 Sep;472(9):2621–2629.

Schenck RC. The dislocated knee. *Instr Course Lect*. 1994;43:127–136.

Sillanpää PJ, Kannus P, Niemi ST, Rolf C et al. Incidence of knee dislocation and concomitant vascular injury requiring surgery: A nationwide study. *J Trauma Acute Care Surg*. 2014 Mar;76(3):715–719.

Stannard JP, Sheils TM, Lopez-Ben RR et al. Vascular injuries in knee dislocations: The role of physical examination in determining the need for arteriography. *J Bone Joint Surg Am*. 2004 May;86(5):910–915.

16

FLOATING KNEE

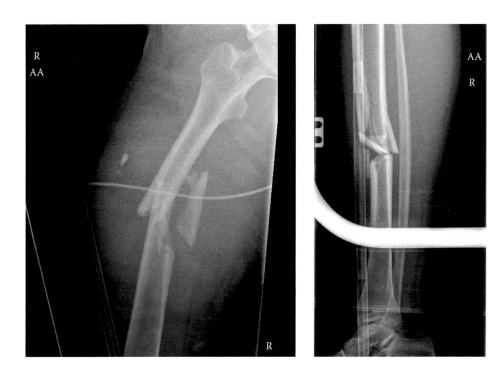

A 55-year-old man is brought to the emergency department after a road traffic accident in which he was the driver of a car in a high-speed collision. He complains of right lower limb pain. The right lower limb is obviously deformed. This is his emergency department radiograph.

1. Describe your initial management in the emergency department.

This patient would be received and managed as a 'trauma call' in the emergency department with assessment and initial management along ATLS guidelines and led by the trauma team leader. The radiograph shows displaced and comminuted fractures of the ipsilateral left femur as well as the tibia with a 'floating knee'. Following the identification and treatment of any immediately life-threatening injuries I would corroborate the history taken so far, complete the physical examination, including a careful assessment of the soft tissues, looking for evidence of any open wound or soft tissue injury and assessing the neurovascular status of the limb.

I would ensure that the patient had adequate analgesia and I would splint the lower limb in an above knee backslab. I would perform a full secondary survey in order to identify any occult injuries once the patient had been stabilised and adequate analgesia given. I would admit the patient for definitive treatment of this injury on a routine trauma list in daytime hours.

2. How would you manage these injuries definitively?

I would advise surgery for these injuries and my preference would be to treat both injuries with reamed intramedullary nailing. This has the advantage of being reasonably quick and efficient and avoids the need for re-draping and re-positioning between procedures. If the patient is positioned supine on a radiolucent table then both fractures can be satisfactorily addressed through the same incision using anterograde nailing for the tibia fracture and retrograde nailing for the femur. This reduces unnecessary movement for the patient who may have other injuries and also reduces surgical time. I would normally plan to stabilise the tibia first as once this has been stabilised it will allow for greater control and traction when performing reduction and intramedullary nail fixation of the femur. In an unstable patient, I would plan to stabilise the femur first regardless in case the patient deteriorates after the first nailing procedure and is unable to tolerate the second. Following surgical stabilisation of both fractures I would perform an examination under anaesthetic of the knee joint in order to identify any ligamentous instability.

FURTHER READING

Lundy DW, Johnson KD. 'Floating knee' injuries: Ipsilateral fractures of the femur and tibia. *J Am Acad Orthop Surg.* 2001 Jul–Aug;9(4):238–245.

17

DISTAL FEMORAL FRACTURE

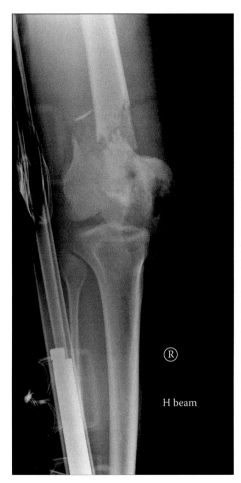
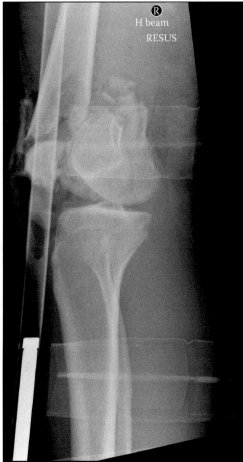

1. **Can you describe the radiographs?**

   This is a highly comminuted distal femoral fracture. There is gas in the soft tissues as well as within the joint, therefore most likely representing an open fracture. The open nature of the injury, plus the degree of comminution and displacement suggests this is an extremely high-energy injury.

2. **The patient is found to have a cold and pale foot in the emergency department. How would you proceed?**

   This is an emergency situation. The patient must be assessed and concurrently resuscitated along ATLS guidelines. This may represent a serious arterial injury although spasm or kinking of the vessel may be responsible. Life or limb-saving intervention may be required emergently.

The neurological status of the limb should be assessed as well as the vascular status examined for warmth, pulses and capillary refill. The limb should be realigned and splinted. Open fracture treatment guidelines should be followed.

Following temporary revascularisation and debridement, I would reassess the wound, soft tissues and the overall patient condition. If suitable for primary fixation I would apply a site-specific, distal femoral plate through a direct lateral approach to stabilise the fracture in a reduced position; otherwise, I would apply a temporary external fixator spanning the knee.

3. What are the features of critical ischaemia in a limb?

The six Ps are indicative of critical ischaemia and should be looked for when performing a vascular status assessment in any fracture. There are three symptoms (pain, paraesthesia, paralysis) and three signs (pale, pulseless, perishingly cold).

4. How would you manage this injury in the operating theatre?

This would be a joint case with involvement of the vascular surgeons and the plastic surgery team due to the open nature of the injury. The primary aim of surgery is to restore blood flow to the affected limb, and this is achieved using an extra-anatomical shunt, therefore minimising the warm ischaemic time. I would then turn my attention to skeletal stability, which is required prior to definitive vascular repair or grafting. My approach with this injury would be to apply standard open fracture treatment with a systematic debridement and washout of the open wound, in addition to washout of the knee joint itself if gas is present on the radiographs. I would apply a site-specific, distal femoral plate through a direct lateral approach to stabilise the fracture in a reduced position.

Once skeletal stability is secured, this allows the vascular surgeons to complete their procedure with a formal repair or graft, without the problem of fracture instability. Where the warm ischaemic time has been greater than 6 hours, compartment syndrome secondary to reperfusion syndrome is likely: prophylactic fasciotomies of the leg (two incision, four compartment) are therefore performed.

5. Given the above information, how would you classify this open fracture?

Using the Gustillo and Anderson open fracture classification, this is a grade 3C: An open fracture with an arterial injury requiring repair.

18

YOUNG FEMORAL FRACTURE

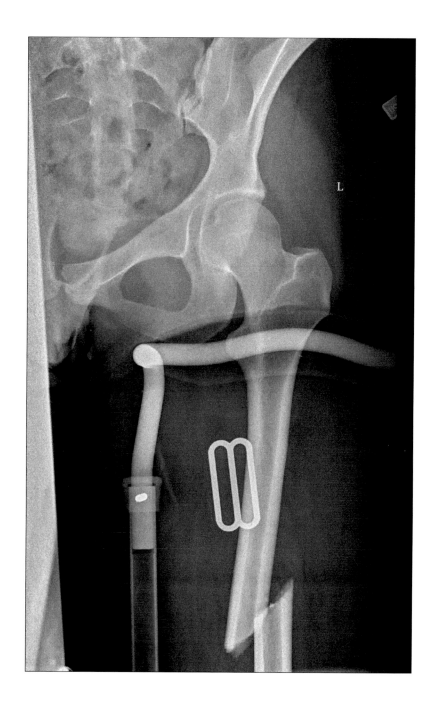

A 29-year-old man is brought into the emergency department after falling off his motorcycle in wet weather. He is treated along ATLS guidelines and his radiograph shows an isolated injury.

1. **Explain what this radiograph shows and describe how you would manage this patient in the emergency department.**

   This is an AP radiograph of the left femur. It shows a displaced midshaft diaphyseal fracture of the femur.

   Following the initial trauma assessment along ATLS guidelines, I would complete a full history and examination including a close examination for any evidence of open wounds and an assessment of the neurological and vascular state of the limb. I would obtain additional imaging to examine the joint above and below in AP and lateral planes. This would either be a trauma CT or additional plain radiographs. I would ensure that the patient had adequate analgesia and I would set up skin traction in the first instance in order to improve analgesia, realign the fracture, reduce blood loss, possibly reduce the risk of fat embolism and reduce any tension on the soft tissues. I would reassess the neurovascular status following this.

   I would examine the patient carefully, performing a secondary survey in order to identify any additional or occult injuries. I would admit the patient to a ward and prepare him for surgery.

2. **When would you choose to take this patient to theatre and what procedure would you perform?**

   In an otherwise stable patient admitted during daylight hours and where they had been or could be appropriately fasted, I would aim to complete surgical treatment ideally on the same day. Should the patient be admitted late in the day, out of hours or where there are complicating factors such as reversible factors or injuries that can be treated to improve outcome, I would delay treatment to the next day routine trauma operating list or when they are best able to tolerate the anaesthetic and surgical insult.

3. **Several hours after surgery, the patient becomes confused, hypoxic and develops a petechial rash over his anterior chest wall. How would you manage and investigate this? What would be in your differential diagnosis?**

   I would assess the patient fully, taking a history, if possible, and perform an examination of the patient. I would look particularly for signs or evidence of fever, tachycardia, chest pain, tachypnoea and agitation. I would take an arterial blood gas sample as well as blood samples for full blood count and urea and electrolytes. I would administer high-flow oxygen and would obtain a chest radiograph and electrocardiogram also. If the patient's level of consciousness was significantly altered or evolving, then I would arrange CT imaging of the head to look for evidence of a missed intracranial bleed. A computer tomography pulmonary angiography (CTPA) would confirm or exclude a pulmonary embolus.

   My differential diagnosis would include fat embolus syndrome, PE, postoperative delirium, intracranial bleed and infection. Of these, fat embolus syndrome seems the most likely to me, but this is a clinical diagnosis and I would need to exclude the more serious conditions I am considering. If the diagnosis is fat embolus syndrome, the treatment is supportive with oxygenation, intravenous fluids, ventilation if required and close monitoring. I would expect the condition to resolve within 72 hours in most cases. Diagnosis of fat embolus syndrome is usually based on at least one major and four minor criteria as set forth by Gurd and Wilson. CTPA is not usually diagnostic but will detect a major pulmonary embolus, and there are some suggestive features on imaging, which in the right clinical context, might support a diagnosis of fat embolus syndrome.

FURTHER READING

Aman J, van Koppenhagen L, Snoek AM, van der Hoeven JG, van der Lely AJ. Cerebral fat embolism after bone fractures. *Lancet.* 2015 Oct 3;386(10001):e16. doi: 10.1016 /S0140-6736(15)60064-2.

Bone LB, Johnson KD, Weigelt J, Scheinberg R. Early versus delayed stabilization of femoral fractures. A prospective randomized study. *J Bone Joint Surg Am.* 1989 Mar;71(3):336–340.

Gandhi RR, Overton TL, Haut ER, Lau B, Vallier HA, Rohs T, Hasenboehler E, Lee JK, Alley D, Watters J, Rogers FB, Shafi S. Optimal timing of femur fracture stabilization in poly-trauma patients: A practice management guideline from the Eastern Association for the Surgery of Trauma. *J Trauma Acute Care Surg.* 2014 Nov;77(5):787–795.

Gray AC, Torrens L, White TO, Carson A, Robinson CM. The cognitive effects of fat embolus syndrome following an isolated femoral shaft fracture. A case report. *J Bone Joint Surg Am.* 2007 May;89(5):1092–1096.

Gurd AR, Wilson RI. The fat embolism syndrome. *J Bone Joint Surg Br.* 1974 Aug;56B(3):408–416.

19

IPSILATERAL FEMORAL NECK AND SHAFT FRACTURE

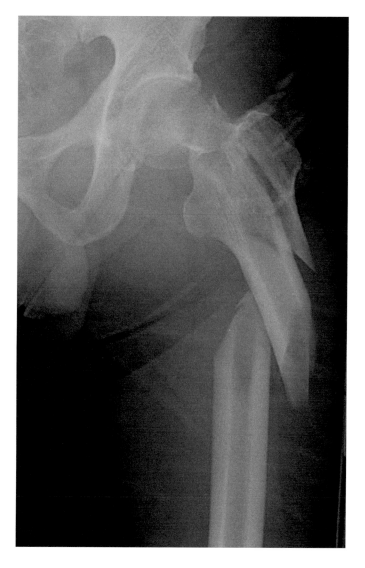

A 20-year-old man is brought to the emergency department following a high-speed road traffic accident in which he was the seat belt–restrained driver of a car. He is treated along ATLS guidelines and is found to have an isolated left lower limb injury as shown in this radiograph.

1. **Describe the appearance in this radiograph.**
   This is an AP radiograph of the left hip and femur. It shows fractures of the ipsilateral neck and shaft of femur, both of which are displaced.

2. **How would you manage and investigate this patient following the initial resuscitation?**

This represents a high-energy injury and this patient would be received and treated in the emergency department along ATLS principles.

I would ensure that the patient is given adequate analgesia. I would perform a full circumferential examination of the limb paying attention to the state of the soft tissues. I would make an assessment of the neurovascular status. I would be careful to look for associated injuries to the knee, ankle and foot. It may be difficult to assess for ligamentous injuries of the knee at this time, but I would remain suspicious. I would ensure that I had good AP and lateral imaging to include the joint above and the joint below.

Assuming this is a closed injury without neurovascular deficit, I would then apply skin traction to the lower leg if the soft tissues would permit this using a 5 kg weight. I would advise operative treatment for this patient and I would prepare the patient for this, including routine blood tests and group and save blood samples and an electrocardiogram, chest radiograph and other perioperative tests as indicated.

3. **What would be your operative plan for this patient? Describe the sequence of surgery.**

This is a high-energy injury. The potential for serious complications is greatest with the femoral neck fracture in this patient and I would address this first. In a consented and appropriately anaesthetised patient, I would position the patient on a fracture table and under traction I would perform a closed anatomic reduction of the femoral neck fracture under image intensification. If required, I would perform an open reduction to achieve this using a Smith–Petersen surgical approach. Once reduced, I would stabilise the femoral neck fracture with three cannulated cancellous large-fragment 6.5 mm screws. For high-grade Pauwels hip fractures with vertically orientated fracture lines, I would choose to use a dynamic hip screw rather than cannulated screws in order to obtain greater stability.

Having achieved rigid fixation of the femoral neck, my preference would be to release the traction, place the patient on a radiolucent table and achieve stable femoral shaft fixation using retrograde intramedullary nailing. This would allow me to avoid potentially interfering with and possibly compromising the proximal fixation to or the residual blood supply of the hip.

4. **What are the potential complications of this injury?**

This is a high-energy injury and the patient could be susceptible to early complications of respiratory compromise, bleeding, compartment syndrome, fat embolus or neurovascular injury. Later, there is the potential for soft tissue complications, wound infection and pulmonary embolus. Specific to this injury there are also the risks of non-union, avascular necrosis of the hip, limb length discrepancy, altered gait and persistent hip or lower limb pain.

FURTHER READING

Boulton CL, Pollak AN. Ipsilateral femoral neck and shaft fractures – Does evidence give us the answer? *Injury.* 2015 Mar;46(3):478–483.

Wolinsky PR, Johnson KD. Ipsilateral femoral neck and shaft fractures. *Clin Orthop Relat Res.* 1995 Sep;(318):81–90.

20

HIP FRACTURE (SUBTROCHANTERIC)

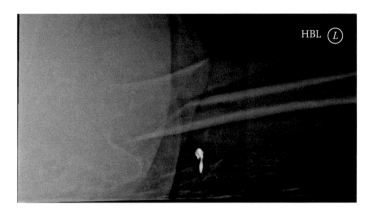

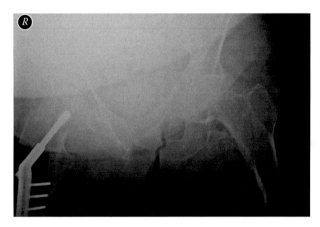

1. **Can you describe the radiographs?**

   These are AP and lateral radiographs of the left hip. The subtrochanteric region extends from the lesser trochanter to 5 cm distal to the lesser trochanter. Therefore, these show a subtrochanteric hip fracture. There is no obvious evidence that this is pathological.

2. **In what position are the fragments lying and why?**

   The proximal fragment is flexed due to the unopposed action of iliopsoas, and abducted due to the glutei. It is also externally rotated due to the action of the short external rotators. If the lesser trochanter is attached to the distal fragment, the classically flexed proximal fragment will not be present.

   The distal fragment is shortened due to the action of the quadriceps and the hamstrings, as well as adducted due to the adductors inserting on the distal fragment.

3. Who gets subtrochanteric hip fractures and how would you classify them?

In the majority of cases, this is a fracture of the elderly. Most are caused by simple falls from a standing height, like all other hip fracture types. However, there is a higher incidence of pathological fractures in this region compared with other types of hip fracture. Patients on bisphosphates are susceptible to transverse fractures in this area, which may show a cortical thickening of the lateral cortex, absence of comminution and a medial spike. If this injury is sustained in a young patient, it is usually the result of a high-energy injury.

These are classified by the Russell–Taylor classification. Type I has no extension into the piriformis fossa, whereas type II does. This is further subdivided into A and B depending on the integrity of the medial buttress. This is a historical classification as type II fractures were treated with a fixed angle device rather than the cephalomedullary nail used today.

4. Would you want any further investigations?

I would want full-length femur views and tailored imaging as indicated after a full history and examination in order to assess for a malignancy.

5. How would you treat this fracture operatively?

I would use a long cephalomedullary nail. In Parker and Handoll's 2010 *Cochrane* review, they found that the use of intramedullary nails may have advantages over fixed angle plates for subtrochanteric and some unstable trochanteric fractures, but admitted that further studies are required to confirm this. More recent studies and meta-analyses have shown that fixation failure and revision surgery is reduced with the use of intramedullary implants for subtrochanteric fractures. The most recent National Institute for Health and Clinical Excellence (NICE) guidelines on hip fractures advise that subtrochanteric fractures are treated with intramedullary nails.

FURTHER READING

Kuzyk PR, Bhandari M, McKee MD et al. Intramedullary versus extramedullary fixation for subtrochanteric femur fractures. *J Orthop Trauma*. 2009;23(6):465–470.

Liu P, Wu X, Shi H et al. Intramedullary versus extramedullary fixation in the management of subtrochanteric femur fractures: A meta-analysis. *Clin Interv Aging*. 2015;10:803–811.

Parker MJ, Handoll HH. Gamma and other cephalocondylic intramedullary nails versus extramedullary implants for extracapsular hip fractures in adults. *Cochrane Database Syst Rev*. 2010 Sep 8;(9):CD000093.

21

PATHOLOGICAL FRACTURE

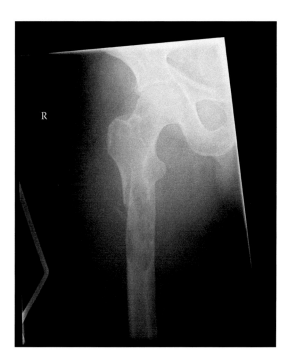

1. **Can you describe the radiograph?**

   This is an AP radiograph of the right hip. There is a pathological fracture of the right femur in the subtrochanteric region of a skeletally mature patient. A lytic area extends from just distal to the lesser trochanter to approximately 10 cm down the femoral shaft. There is cortical destruction and a relatively broad zone of transition. The matrix of the lesion is predominantly lytic. There are no other obvious areas of abnormal bone on the visualised femur and pelvis although plain radiographs are often unreliable as a measure of cortical destruction. Most studies state that at least 30% of bone destruction must take place prior to any changes being visible.

2. **What is your differential diagnosis?**

   The differential diagnosis is dependent on the age of the patient. I would be highly suspicious of metastasis when considering a lytic lesion of bone in a patient over the age of 40, particularly in the proximal femur. In a younger patient, the differential diagnosis would include a variety of lesions which present with lysis (listed below).

3. **The patient in question is 65 years old. How would you proceed if presented with this radiograph?**

   The patient has a fractured femur with a potential for blood loss and significant pain. I would ensure they are stable haemodynamically and have received appropriate analgesia prior to moving on to a full history and examination. Since the main differential diagnosis is of metastasis, I would conduct a full history and examination, concentrating on identifying the primary tumour. As the main sources for a primary tumour are breast, bronchus, thyroid, kidney and prostate, I would focus my history and examination on these areas.

Following a full history and examination, I would organise a full set of blood tests including FBC, U&Es, LFTs, TFTs, bone profiling (alkaline phosphatase, calcium and albumin), CRP, ESR, and tumour markers, in addition to a myeloma screen (which should include urine electrophoresis to look for Bence Jones protein). In terms of imaging, I would want plain radiographs of the rest of the femur with orthogonal views. I would organise a CT of the chest, abdomen and pelvis to look for a primary tumour, as well as a bone scan to look for other skeletal deposits. An MRI scan of the lesion would also be helpful. Following rapid investigation, the patient should be discussed with the local tumour service to discuss management and further investigation, which will include biopsy in most cases.

Biopsy should be performed by the tumour surgeon who will ultimately be treating the pathological fracture. It is particularly useful where there is diagnostic doubt or, in a solitary bone lesion, where there may be a chance for curative treatment. It is probably superfluous to requirements if the diagnosis is disseminated metastatic malignancy to bone.

4. **What are the management principles when dealing with any pathological fracture?**
The aims of surgery with any pathological fracture are ideally to ensure a single operation for the patient to restore function and remove pain. It should allow immediate and full weight bearing, carry minimal morbidity, deal with all the metastatic disease within that bone and minimise time spent in hospital. Although pathological fractures can unite, there is a much higher rate of non-union as well as a longer time to union.

When considering treatment options, it is also pertinent to ascertain a life expectancy for the patient in conjunction with the oncologists.

The Scandinavian Sarcoma Group produced a scoring system to estimate survival after bone metastases. It allows clinicians to estimate survival and subsequently tailor treatments for pathological fractures.

5. **When dealing with a pathological lesion within a bone, how does one estimate the risk of fracture?**
As a rule of thumb, where 50% of a single cortex of a long bone (in any radiological view) has been destroyed, patients are at significant risk of pathological fracture. In addition, avulsion of the lesser trochanter is an indication of imminent hip fracture.

The Mirels score is frequently used to calculate the risk of fracture in long bones. Mirels proposed a scoring system based on four characteristics: (1) site of lesion; (2) nature of lesion; (3) size of lesion; and (4) pain. All the features were assigned progressive scores ranging from 1 to 3, and the current recommendation from the BOA/BOOS guidelines is that a score of 9 or greater warrants prophylactic fixation prior to radiotherapy.

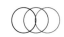
Mnemonics for Bone Lesions

LYTIC – FOGMACHINES	*SCLEROTIC* – 'Surgical sieve' VITAMIN CD
F: Fibrous dysplasia or fibrous cortical defect (FCD)	Vascular: Haemangiomas, bony infarcts
O: Osteoblastoma	Infection: Chronic osteomyelitis
G: Giant cell tumour (GCT)	Trauma: Stress fractures/healing fractures
M: Metastasis/myeloma	Autoimmune
A: Aneurysmal bone cyst (ABC)	Metabolic: Hyperparathyroidism, Paget's disease
C: Chondroblastoma or chondromyxoid fibroma	Inflammatory/Idiopathic
H: Hyperparathyroidism (brown tumour)	Neoplastic:
I: Infection (osteomyelitis)	• Primary – Osteoma, Osteosarcoma
N: Non-ossifying fibroma (NOF)	• Metastatic – Prostate and breast, most commonly
E: Enchondroma or eosinophilic granuloma (EG)	Congenital: Bone islands, Osteopoikilosis, Osteopetrosis, Pyknodysostosis
S: Simple (unicameral) bone cyst	Drugs: Vitamin D, fluoride, lead poisoning

FURTHER READING

British Orthopaedic Oncology Society & British Orthopaedic Association. *Metastatic Bone Disease: A Guide to Good Practice*. 2015 revision.

Mirels H. Metastatic disease in long bones: A proposed scoring system for diagnosing impending pathologic fractures. 1989. *Clin Orthop Relat Res.* 2003 Oct;(415 Suppl):S4–13.

Ratasvuori MI, Wedin R, Keller J, Nottrott M et al. Insight opinion to surgically treated metastatic bone disease: Scandinavian Sarcoma Group Skeletal Metastasis Registry report of 1195 operated skeletal metastasis. *Surg Oncol.* 2013 Jun;22(2):132–138.

22

INTRACAPSULAR HIP FRACTURE YOUNG PATIENT

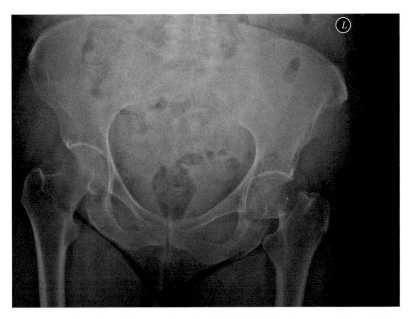

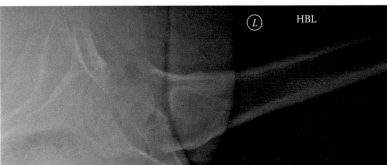

These are the radiographs for a 36-year-old cyclist hit by a car. It is an isolated injury.

1. **Describe the x-rays.**
   These are AP and lateral radiographs of the left hip showing a displaced intracapsular fracture of the neck of the femur.

2. **Describe the blood supply to the femoral head and explain why this is important.**
   The blood supply to the femoral head comes from three groups of vessels. First, an extracapsular arterial ring at the base of the femoral neck formed from the medial and lateral circumflex femoral arteries. Ascending arterial vessels arising from the extraarticular ring and passing proximally on the femoral neck form a retinacular

supply in close proximity to the bony surface of the femoral neck. Second, an arterial supply in the ligament of Teres, which may atrophy over time and therefore becomes less important with age although there is often some persistent supply. Finally, the femoral head also has an intraosseous blood from nutrient blood vessels.

Therefore, in a femoral neck fracture, the intraosseous blood supply to the femoral head is disrupted and the remaining supply may be provided only by the remaining retinacular vessels. Increasing displacement of the fracture may indicate increasing energy of injury and likelihood of disruption to these vessels so that displaced femoral neck fractures have a greater chance of rendering the femoral head avascular than undisplaced fractures.

3. How would you manage this injury and patient?

A femoral neck fracture in a young patient often represents a high-energy injury and the patient should be treated along ATLS principles. Assuming this is an isolated injury, I would plan to treat the hip fracture urgently to try to minimise the period of ischaemia to the femoral head. In a young patient with reasonable bone quality, conserving the native femoral head avoids the risks and long-term consequences of arthroplasty. There is debate as to whether the use of a formal capsulotomy might reduce the local tamponade effect of the haematoma on the femoral head and the resulting risk of avascular necrosis. There is no good evidence to support this and it is not something that I would do routinely. I would choose to manage this patient with closed reduction of the fracture and internal fixation. There is debate as to whether cannulated screws or a sliding hip screw device and plate provide ideal fixation. In a young patient I would choose to use a sliding hip screw because it resists shear forces better, particularly in more vertical (Pauwel 3) fracture types. I would use a standard lateral approach if the fracture reduced satisfactorily and easily with a closed approach. If closed reduction is difficult or unsatisfactory, I would proceed to an open reduction using the anterolateral Watson–Jones approach. This would allow me to visualise and adjust the fracture reduction, to temporarily stabilise the fracture with K-wires to avoid subsequent rotation and to fix the fracture with a sliding hip screw all through the same incision. This also gives me the option of placing an additional cannulated anti-rotation screw over the initial K-wire for additional rotational stability.

4. Would you impose any limitations on the patient, how long would you follow them up for and what would you tell them about the relative merits and risks of the different treatment options?

I would tell the patient that this is a serious injury with potential long-term consequences. Any form of hip fracture surgery carries risks including scar, infection, DVT, and neurovascular injury. The management choice is mainly whether to fix or replace the fracture. My advice would be that in a young, active patient with relatively high demands, fixing the fracture rather than performing a form of replacement surgery conserves the patient's own bone and avoids the complications associated with arthroplasty such as dislocation, bearing wear and periprosthetic fracture. Fracture fixation does carry risks of non-union as well as painful post-traumatic arthritis, failure of fixation and avascular necrosis. With these in mind, I would undertake urgent surgery, up until the early hours of the same evening of presentation or first thing the next day, but not in the middle of the night. I would limit the patient to toe-touch weight bearing for 6 weeks postoperatively and I would follow the patient up clinically and radiographically for 2 years to identify signs of avascular necrosis. Although there is limited evidence for some of these measures, they aim to minimise the risk of early loss of fixation and avascular necrosis.

FURTHER READING

Harper WM, Barnes MR, Gregg PJ. Femoral head blood flow in femoral neck fractures. An analysis using intra-osseous pressure measurement. *J Bone Joint Surg Br.* 1991 Jan;73(1):73–75.

Jain R, Koo M, Kreder HJ, Schemitsch EH, Davey JR, Mahomed NN. Comparison of early and delayed fixation of subcapital hip fractures in patients sixty years of age or less. *J Bone Joint Surg Am.* 2002 Sep;84-A(9):1605–1612.

Ly TV, Swiontkowski MF. Treatment of femoral neck fractures in young adults. *J Bone Joint Surg Am.* 2008 Oct;90(10):2254–2266.

Upadhyay A, Jain P, Mishra P, Maini L, Gautum VK, Dhaon BK. Delayed internal fixation of fractures of the neck of the femur in young adults. A prospective, randomised study comparing closed and open reduction. *J Bone Joint Surg Br.* 2004 Sep;86(7):1035–1040.

Zielinski SM, Keijsers NL, Praet SF, Heetveld MJ, Bhandari M, Wilssens JP, Patka P, Van Lieshout EM; FAITH Trial Investigators. Functional outcome after successful internal fixation versus salvage arthroplasty of patients with a femoral neck fracture. *J Orthop Trauma.* 2014 Dec;28(12):e273–e280.

23

HIP FRACTURE

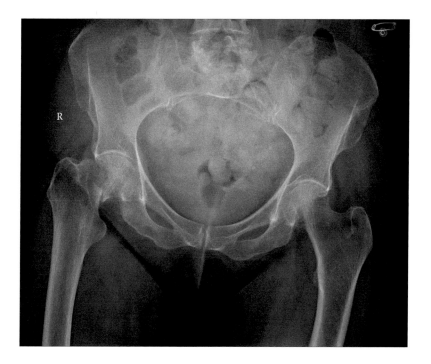

This 79-year-old woman fell in the street after getting off the bus, sustaining the above injury.

1. **Can you describe the radiograph, and how would you classify this fracture?**
   This is an AP radiograph of both hips showing a displaced intracapsular hip fracture on the right side. This can be classified according to the Garden classification but, in practice, I would describe it as undisplaced or displaced as this is what would determine my management. This radiograph in particular shows a displaced intra-capsular hip fracture.

2. **What is the blood supply to the femoral head?**
   The vascular supply to the femoral head arises from three sources. One of these is the ligamentum teres: this contains a branch of the obturator artery which, in adults, provides a negligible source of blood supply to the femoral head, in contrast to children.

   The second source is from the medullary canal, which is of course disrupted in a femoral neck fracture.

   The third source is from the lateral and medial circumflex femoral arteries, which are branches of the profunda femoris artery. The medial circumflex femoral artery provides a larger proportion of blood supply than its lateral counterpart. These form a vascular anastamosis at the base of the capsule and, from this, retinacular vessels run along the femoral neck underneath the capsule to supply the femoral head. These are potentially disrupted in displaced intracapsular hip fractures.

3. **What information would you want to gather from taking a history?**
Assuming this is an isolated injury and the patient has been given suitable analgesia, I would like to take a full history in order to rule out a medical cause for her fall and if she is suitable for a total hip replacement or best managed with a hemiarthroplasty.

To determine if a medical cause was responsible for her fall, I would start with a history regarding preceding symptoms, such as chest pain, palpitations, dizziness, weakness or SOB, and any history of previous falls. I would take a full systematic enquiry to look for evidence of infection, particular urinary and respiratory infections. Regarding a pathological fracture, I would ask about constitutional symptoms of malignancy (weight loss, loss of appetite, night sweats) and preceding hip pain prior to the fall.

I would go on to ask about her past medical history, drug history (particularly warfarin), social history, including level of mobility and mobility aids, fall risks as well as a mental state examination. I would perform a DVT risk assessment and consider whether this patient is at risk of further fragility fractures and should have investigation to determine bone quality and treatment if required.

4. **What examination and investigations would you perform in the emergency department, and what initial treatments would you commence?**
Examination would consist of a full set of observations and confirmation of pain on movement of the affected limb in a gentle fashion. I would assess the neurovascular status of the leg and examine the skin around the planned incision site. I would assess for other injuries, common sites including the distal radius and proximal humerus, as well as perform a cardiovascular and respiratory examination.

Routine bloods would include FBC, U&Es and group and save, plus a coagulation screen if indicated.

A chest radiograph is generally indicated in all elderly patients with a hip fracture +/– full-length femur views depending on local protocols. An ECG would also be performed in the emergency department.

IV fluids should be initiated as patients are generally dehydrated and oral intake will be minimal in the ward owing to pain +/– confusion.

To be suitable for a THR, patients should be medically fit for a longer operation with more blood loss, must be cognitively intact in order to implement standard hip precautions and should be independent ambulators who will benefit from the improved patient reported outcomes. There is good evidence to support the use of THR in the fit elderly patient. This should be discussed with the patient in order to gain informed consent, making sure to mention a slightly increased rate of dislocation compared to hemiarthroplasty.

All patients should ideally be admitted to a dedicated hip fracture ward within 4 hours of arrival in A&E and should be seen both pre- and postoperatively by an orthogeriatrician. Their operation should be performed within 48 hours in order to prevent a worse outcome unless there is a readily reversible medical problem.

5. **Do you know of any guidelines that direct your management of hip fracture patients?**
Several guidelines exist to provide an overview of the available evidence and guide best practise when treating hip fractures. These include the Scottish Intercollegiate

Guidelines Network (SIGN), National Institute for Health and Clinical Excellence (NICE) and British Orthopaedic Association Standards for Trauma (BOAST) guidelines.

Links to these guidelines are as follows:

- SIGN, http://www.sign.ac.uk/guidelines/fulltext/111/
- NICE, https://www.nice.org.uk/guidance/cg124
- BOAST, http://www.boa.ac.uk/publications/boa-standards-trauma-boasts/

FURTHER READING

Moja L, Piatti A, Pecoraro V, Ricci C, Virgili G, Salanti G, Germagnoli L, Liberati A, Banfi G. Timing matters in hip fracture surgery: Patients operated within 48 hours have better outcomes. A meta-analysis and meta-regression of over 190,000 patients. *PLoS One.* 2012;7(10):e46175.

24

PERIPROSTHETIC FRACTURE

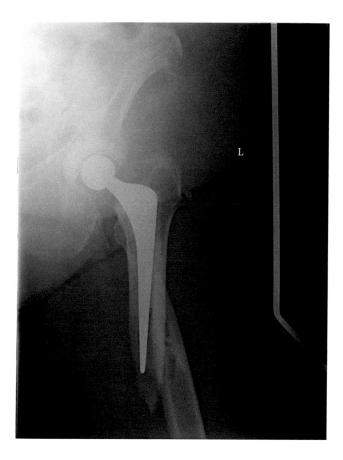

A 68-year-old woman is brought to the emergency department after falling in the shower. Her radiograph is above.

1. **Describe the appearances in this radiograph.**

   This is an AP radiograph of the left hip and femur. It shows a cemented total hip replacement that looks well-fixed and an associated periprosthetic fracture of the femur at the level of the tip of the prosthesis. I would obtain additional radiographs so that I have adequate AP and lateral imaging for the hip and the whole femur, and I would classify this using the Vancouver system of classification proposed by Duncan and Masri, although I know that Duncan has proposed an update to this classification system, the unified classification system.

   Based on the imaging available, I believe that this is a type B-1 fracture.

2. **How would you manage and investigate this patient?**

   I would undertake a full history and examination of this patient. These injuries are more common in frail elderly patients and I would pay particular attention to the cause of the fall, co-morbidities, pre-injury function and satisfaction with the hip replacement and also any suggestion of wound problems or infection following the original surgery. I would send routine blood samples for full blood count, serum electrolytes and a sample for group and save. I believe this fracture would be best treated operatively. I would also send samples for CRP and ESR as part of a general screen for infection. I would prepare the patient for theatre, obtaining an electro-cardiogram and chest x-ray if necessary based on the history and clinical findings. I would also ensure that this patient is assessed for her risk of fragility fractures with a falls assessment and dual energy x-ray absorptiometry (DEXA) scan. In my unit this is part of a detailed assessment from the orthogeriatric service.

3. **What are the treatment options for this patient?**

This can be treated with operative or non-operative management. Non-operative management with traction is possible as the implant is well-fixed as long as alignment is maintained, but this will leave the patient exposed to all the risks of prolonged recumbency.

I would advise operative management. I would choose to use an open sub-vastus approach to reduce the fracture and to temporarily stabilise it with cerclage wires. This would also allow me to take perioperative tissue samples for microbiology. I would choose to apply a locking plate (LC-DCP) to the lateral aspect of the femur using several unicortical screws proximally so as not violate the cement mantle of the femoral stem and using bicortical screws more distally. I would reposition or completely replace the temporising cerclage wires so that two or three wires provide additional stability to the proximal construct where the screw fixation is unicortical. In addition, if there is an obvious cortical defect or marked comminution I would use a femoral cortical strut allograft which I would lay on the anterior aspect of the femur so that it bypasses the defect or area of comminution by at least two cortical widths. I would incorporate this into the cerclage wire fixation.

The evidence for the use of locking plates, cerclage wires or onlay cortical strut grafts is limited to case series. There is, however, some good evidence that where the fracture pattern is a B-2 type, with a loose femoral implant, the results of arthroplasty are superior to those of operative fixation.

FURTHER READING

Dehghan N, McKee MD, Nauth A, Ristevski B, Schemitsch EH. Surgical fixation of Vancouver type B1 periprosthetic femur fractures: A systematic review. *J Orthop Trauma.* 2014 Dec;28(12):721–727.

Duncan CP. The Unified Classification System (UCS): Improving our understanding of periprosthetic fractures. *Bone Joint J.* 2014;96-B:713–716.

Masri BA, Meek RM, Duncan CP. Periprosthetic fractures evaluation and treatment. *Clin Orthop Relat Res.* 2004 Mar;(420):80–95. Review.

25

POSTERIOR DISLOCATION OF THE HIP

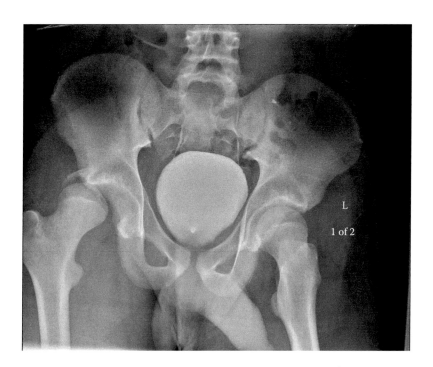

1. **What does this radiograph show and how would you manage this in the emergency department?**

   This is an AP radiograph of the pelvis, demonstrating a posterior fracture-dislocation of the hip. There is an associated fracture of the posterior wall of the acetabulum. As this is a high-energy injury, I would assess and manage the patient as per ATLS guidelines. I would assess the neurovascular status of the limb, particularly the sciatic nerve, and provide analgesia. The patient requires emergent reduction of the hip in order to reduce tension on the sciatic nerve and reduce the risk of AVN, and I would perform this in theatre to ensure the patient can be fully anaesthetised with general anaesthesia and muscle relaxant in order to minimise trauma to the femoral head when performing the reduction. Following reduction and my assessment of the stable range, I would expect the hip to be unstable in flexion, so I would immobilise the patient in a soft Thackray knee splint to limit hip flexion.

2. **Describe how you perform a closed reduction?**

   I would perform Bigelow's manoeuvre. This requires an assistant to stabilise the pelvis via the anterior superior iliac spines. I would then apply traction, adduction and internal rotation. Reduction is usually associated with an audible 'clunk' and would be confirmed using the image intensifier. I would then assess stability of the hip as this may determine the need for further operative intervention. I would do this under image intensifier as I would not want to re-dislocate the hip and risk further cartilage damage.

3. **What would your postoperative management consist of following a closed reduction of the hip?**

I would confirm and record the stable range of movement of the hip once reduced. I would assess the neurovascular status of the patient in theatre recovery, particularly the sciatic nerve. I would want to obtain a CT scan of the hip urgently in order to rule out any intra-articular bony fragments in addition to obtaining a better appreciation of the posterior wall fracture.

4. **What are the indications for fixing a posterior wall fracture in association with a hip dislocation?**

Surgery is required if there is instability of the hip (best confirmed in theatre following closed reduction) or a lack of joint congruity.

5. **How would you proceed if the hip would not reduce closed?**

Failed closed reduction necessitates an open reduction through a posterior approach to the hip, extended proximally into a Kocher–Langenbeck approach if there was a posterior wall fracture in need of fixation. I would take particular care not to damage the sciatic nerve as it may be displaced due to the dislocated hip. I would be careful to stay away from quadratus femoris in order to avoid damage to the medial circumflex femoral artery (MCFA), and would incise the short external rotators at least 1.5 cm from their insertions to again avoid damage to the MCFA.

6. **What would you use to fix the posterior wall fracture?**

There are several constructs available depending on the size of the fragment and the degree of comminution. I would assess the fragment intraoperatively and then use either large fragment lag screws +/− buttress plate using a 3.5 mm reconstruction plate, or create a hook plate by breaking a small fragment one-third tubular plate through a hole at the tip and bending the ends such that the hooks are perpendicular to the plate.

7. **What clinical and radiographic findings would you see in an anterior dislocation of the hip, and what is the usual mechanism of injury for this?**

Anterior dislocations of the hip are rare and they occur when the hip is in a position of abduction and external rotation. Clinically, the leg may be shortened and generally held in flexion, abduction and external rotation, compared to a posterior dislocation where the leg is held in flexion, adduction and internal rotation.

FURTHER READING

Moed BR, Ajibade DA, Israel H. Computed tomography as a predictor of hip stability status in posterior wall fractures of the acetabulum. *J Orthop Trauma*. 2009 Jan;23(1):7–15.

Tornetta P III. Non-operative management of acetabular fractures. The use of dynamic stress views. *J Bone Joint Surg Br*. 1999 Jan;81(1):67–70.

26

ACETABULUM FRACTURE

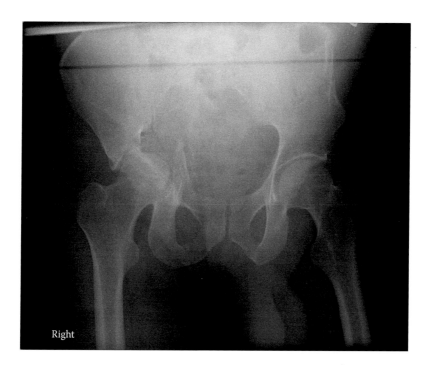

Right

A 25-year-old man has been involved in a high-speed road traffic accident.

1. What do these radiographs show and how would you manage this?

These radiographs show a grossly displaced acetabular fracture on the right side. There is disruption of the iliopectineal line as well as the ilioischial line and dome of the acetabulum. This is a high-energy injury, and the possibility of other life-threatening injuries must be actively searched for using an ATLS approach to systematic diagnosis and concurrent management in the emergency department.

With regard to the acetabular fracture itself, an assessment should be made of the skin to rule out an open fracture, a Morel–Lavallée lesion, or any wounds which may interfere with planned surgical incisions. I would also perform a full neurovascular assessment of the affected limb and wish to exclude urogenital injuries. Unlike pelvic fractures, there is unlikely to be a life-threatening haemorrhage with an isolated acetabular fracture, and pelvic binders would not be indicated.

2. What additional radiographs might give you a better appreciation of the bony injury, and what is the importance of these?

Two additional radiographs may be utilised to improve the preoperative understanding of the acetabular fracture. These are Judet views, which are composed of two projections: First, the iliac oblique for assessment of the posterior column and anterior wall; second, the obturator oblique view for the anterior column and posterior wall.

Although centres where patients are treated for these injuries will have access to modern CT scanning, these views have that advantage that can be achieved with the image intensifier in the operating theatre and are therefore a useful pre- and perioperative adjunct to fixation.

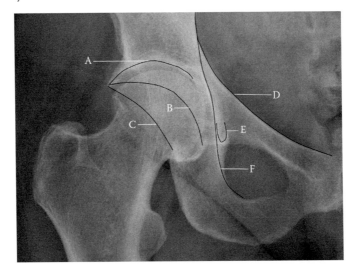

3. **Can you name the labelled areas of the plain AP radiograph of the pelvis?**
   A – Acetabular dome/roof
   B – Anterior wall
   C – Posterior wall
   D – Iliopectineal line (represents the anterior column)
   E – Tear drop
   F – Ilioischial line (represents the posterior column)

4. **What is the 'tear drop'?**
   The pelvic tear drop results from the end-on projection of a bony ridge running along the floor of the acetabulum.

   It is formed laterally by the confluence of subchondral bone at the floor of the acetabular fossa (also known as the cotyloid fossa) and medially by the anterior flat portion of quadrilateral plate.

   It represents the true floor of the acetabulum and is frequently used for preoperative planning in hip arthroplasty.

5. **What anatomical structures make up the anterior and posterior columns of the acetabulum?**
   Anterior column:
   - Anterior iliac wing
   - Anterior wall and dome
   - Iliopectineal eminence
   - Superior pubic ramus

   Posterior column:
   - Quadrilateral plate
   - Posterior wall and dome
   - Ischial tuberosity
   - Greater/lesser sciatic notches

6. How are acetabular fractures classified and what are the most common fracture patterns?

The most commonly referred to classification systems is the Judet and Letournel classification. This divides acetabular fractures into five 'elementary' types and five 'associated' fracture patterns. The elementary fractures are named as such owing to the involvement of only one element of pelvic anatomy. The most common acetabular fracture is an elementary fracture of the posterior wall. Others include the anterior column, anterior wall, posterior column and transverse fracture pattern.

Associated fractures imply the presence of two or more of the elementary fracture patterns. The most common of these are the (1) transverse/posterior wall fracture and (2) the both column fracture, where there is complete dissociation of the articular surface from the inonimate bone. The both column fracture can be diagnosed in the presence of a 'spur sign', which is produced by a triangular fragment of iliac bone that remains attached to the sacroiliac joint but is separated from the fractured acetabulum. This spur is exposed when the fractured acetabular columns are displaced medially in a both column fracture. It is best seen on the obturator oblique view or on a CT scanning of the pelvis, although it can occasionally be seen on a plain AP radiograph.

7. What are the complications of operative treatment of acetabular fractures?

I would divide these into local or systemic and early or late complications.

Early local complications would include sciatic nerve injury (may be injured preoperatively), bleeding and infection – particularly in the context of a Morel–Lavallée lesion.

Early systemic complications would include venous thromboembolism, chest infection, urinary infection and other medical complications related to high-energy injuries, for example, ARDS, SIRS, MODS.

Late local complications would include mal-union, non-union, post-traumatic arthritis and AVN, in addition to ongoing pain and stiffness. Heterotopic ossification is also a well-recognised complication of acetabular surgery.

27

PELVIC FRACTURE

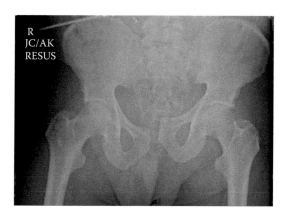

1. **What does this radiograph show, and how would you manage this?**

   This radiograph shows a vertical shear type injury to the pelvis. This is typically the result of a high-energy injury, such as a road traffic accident or a fall from heights, and the possibility of other life-threatening injuries must be actively searched for using an ATLS approach to systematic diagnosis and management.

2. **What would you expect to find on examination?**

   As part of the ATLS assessment it is possible that embarrassment to any and several body systems might be identified during the concurrent assessment and resuscitation of the patient. If there is an isolated injury to the pelvis, the patient may very well be distressed due to pain and potentially confused or agitated due to haemorrhagic shock. Additionally, there may be tachypnoea, tachycardia and hypotension.

   On inspection, there may be an apparent leg length discrepancy in a vertical shear fracture where one hemipelvis is displaced proximally.

   With regard to urogenital and rectal examinations, I would inspect for blood at the urethral meatus, as well as scrotal/labial/perineal haematoma, which may suggest significant urological trauma.

   I would also inspect the state of the soft tissues in order to rule out an open fracture and to exclude a Morel–Lavallée lesion.

   Moving onto palpation, a vaginal examination and rectal examination (in the supine position) to rule out a surreptitious open fracture is mandatory. I would palpate for a high-riding prostate (another sign of significant urethral injury) and anal tone/sensation to assess the sacral nerve roots.

   I would also perform a full neurovascular examination of the lower limbs.

   I would advise against 'springing' the pelvis as a method of diagnosing a pelvic fracture as this is painful, may disrupt a clot which is preventing torrential haemorrhage and is superfluous in the presence of an AP pelvic radiograph taken as part of a trauma series.

3. **In the absence of a CT, what additional radiographs might give you a better appreciation of the bony injury, and how would you obtain these?**

Two views are utilised to better visualise the pelvic ring. Although rarely used for diagnostic purposes given the ready access to modern CT scanning, these are the views that can be achieved with an image intensifier in theatre.

The first of these is an inlet view: The x-ray beam is angled approximately 45 degrees caudal, and an adequate image is obtained when S1 overlaps S2. This view is ideal for diagnosing widening of the SI joints, sacral ala impaction fractures, subtle pubic symphyseal injuries, as well as internal/external rotation or anterior/posterior translation of a hemipelvis.

The second is the outlet view: To obtain this, the x-ray beam is angled approximately 45 degrees cephalad. An adequate image is obtained when the pubic symphysis overlies the S2 body. Conversely, this is ideal for visualising vertical translation of a hemipelvis, as well as flexion/extension of a hemipelvis. As this is a true AP radiograph of the sacrum, it is ideal for diagnosing sacral fractures and their location in relation to the foramina.

4. **How would you classify pelvic fractures?**

I would classify these using the Young and Burgess classification of pelvic fractures. This define pelvic fractures into three categories, with subtypes of each. The categories are I – anterior posterior compression (APC); II – lateral compression (LC); and III – vertical shear (VS).

- APC I – Pubic symphysis widening <2.5 cm. This can be difficult to assess in the presence of a pelvic binder however. Can be managed conservatively.
- APC II – Pubic symphysis widening >2.5 cm. There has been disruption of the sacrospinous and sacrotuberous ligaments, as well as the anterior SI ligaments. The strong posterior SI ligaments remain intact and subsequently there is no loss of vertical stability.
- APC III – As per APC II but with disruption of the strong posterior SI ligaments. This results in loss of vertical stability and is indistinguishable from a vertical shear injury radiographically.
- LC I – Oblique or transverse pubic rami fractures, in addition to crush/compression fracture of the ipsilateral sacral ala.
- LC II – In addition to the pubic rami fractures, there is a characteristic 'crescent' fracture of the iliac wing.
- LC III – There is an ipsilateral lateral compression injury and a contralateral open book injury, known as a 'windswept pelvis'.
- VS – There is complete discontinuity of the sacral attachment to the lower limb. The posterior sacral ring may fail through the SI joint, the sacrum, or the ilium.

5. **What are the common sources of bleeding in a pelvic fracture?**

The most common source of bleeding (approximately 80%) in pelvic fractures is secondary to a shearing injury to the thin-walled posterior venous plexus. Fractures may result in clinically significant blood loss from cancellous bone surfaces.

Arterial injury is a less common source but the arteries most frequently implicated include the superior gluteal artery (APC pattern), the internal pudendal artery (LC pattern) and the obturator artery (LC pattern).

Although there are several specific sites for bleeding in association with pelvic fractures, one must remain vigilant for other sources associated with the high-energy mechanism of injury (intra-abdominal, intra-thoracic, limbs).

28

PELVIC FRACTURE

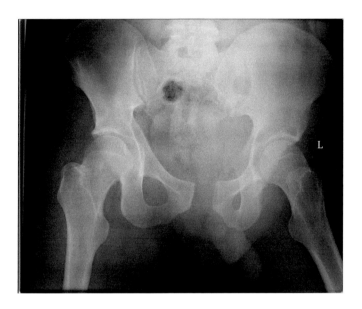

1. **What does this radiograph show and how would you classify this injury?**
   This is an AP radiograph of the pelvis. It shoes an APC II fracture as per the Young and Burgess classification of pelvic fractures. The pubic symphysis has been disrupted, as well as the sacrotuberous, sacrospinous and anterior SI joint ligaments. The strong posterior SI ligaments appear intact as the left hemipelvis seems to have maintained vertical stability, distinguishing it from an APC III or vertical shear type injury.

2. **What signs would you look for to rule out a urological injury and how would you manage a suspected urethral injury in conjunction with this pelvic fracture?**
   A high-riding prostate, blood at the urethral meatus or scrotal/labial/perineal haematoma may suggest significant urological trauma. This requires caution but does allow for a single, gentle attempt at urethral catheterisation. If the catheter does not pass or drains blood, the balloon must not be inflated. The catheter should be withdrawn and a retrograde urethrogram should be performed. Any concerns regarding urological injury must be discussed with the urology service.

   Any suspected urethral injuries in females and children should be discussed with the urology service urgently.

   If a urethral catheter cannot be passed, a suprapubic catheter is required. However, this can alter the approaches available for fracture fixation due to their predilection for infection and must therefore be placed with caution and should only be sited by the urologists after discussion with the pelvic fracture service.

A bladder rupture must be considered in the presence of haematuria. This can be confirmed with a cystogram. If a bladder rupture is identified, these can be either intraperitoneal or extraperitoneal. Intraperitoneal rupture requires emergency laparotomy and direct repair. Although extraperitoneal rupture can be treated by catheter drainage alone, in the presence of an unstable pelvic fracture, it is now recommended that fracture fixation is performed along with a primary repair of the bladder.

With regard to urethral injuries in men, the majority of these are treated with delayed repair at 3 months. However, there are several indications for early repair which will be determined by the local urological service.

3. **What are the different responses to resuscitation in a trauma patient with a pelvic fracture, and how will this determine your immediate management?**
All patients should have an ATLS approach to management and resuscitation as well as a pelvic binder in place, with most modern resuscitation protocols recommending the early appropriate use of blood products for fluid resuscitation in the setting of ongoing haemorrhage. This is administered in a ratio of 1:1:1 ratio of red blood cells: platelets: fresh frozen plasma. Patients are then classified as

- Responders: These patients respond quickly and fully to fluid resuscitation, with no deterioration in their vital signs. These patients lost blood at the time of injury but have no/minimal active bleeding at present.
- Partial responders: These patients respond to resuscitation attempts and fluid (blood) replacement, but their vital signs subsequently deteriorate when this replacement is stopped. This demonstrates continuing, although not catastrophic, haemorrhage.
- Non-responders: These patients remain shocked (tachycardic and hypotensive) despite appropriate fluid (blood) resuscitation as above. This generally indicates rapid and extensive haemorrhage.

If a patient is a responder to resuscitation, they can be managed according to the stability of the pelvic ring. If unstable, they can be managed for planned fixation; if stable, they can be managed conservatively.

Non-responders are usually too unwell to undergo a CT scan. If the pelvic ring is stable, this ongoing haemorrhage is unlikely to be due to pelvic pathology. One should consider a laparotomy +/– thoracotomy as clinically indicated.

Greater than 80% of life-threatening bleeding in an unstable pelvic fracture is due to the posteriorly sited venous plexus. Angiography is therefore less likely to help the patient than pelvic packing in the time-critical setting as it takes longer to perform, leading to increased blood loss.

There is controversy regarding the management of partial responders. Most centres would advocate a judicious approach with Focused Assessment with Sonography for Trauma (FAST) scans +/– CT angiogram +/– embolisation in order to identify the source of bleeding and targeted surgery or interventional radiology depending on the findings. It should be noted that there is a false negative rate associated with FAST scans and diagnostic periteoneal lavage (DPL).

4. **How would you perform a retrograde urethrogram?**
   I would place an x-ray plate under the pelvis and prepare 20 millilitres of diluted IV contrast (10 ml contrast + 10 ml saline). Next, a small Foley catheter is gently inserted into the urethra and the balloon carefully inflated at the urethral meatus and held in place as the contrast is injected. An AP pelvic radiograph is then taken, in addition to a lateral view, if possible.

FURTHER READING

British Orthopaedic Association Audit Standard for Trauma (BOAST). BOAST 14: The management of urological trauma associated with pelvic fractures. 2016. Accessed 1 September 2016 from https://www.boa.ac.uk/wp-content/uploads/2016/09/BOAST-14 -Urological-Injuries.pdf.

National Institute for Health and Clinical Excellence (NICE). Major trauma: Assessment and initial management. 2016. Accessed 1 May 2016 from https://www.nice.org.uk/guidance /ng39.

SECTION II
SPINE AND UPPER LIMB TRAUMA

29

BILATERAL CERVICAL FACET DISLOCATION

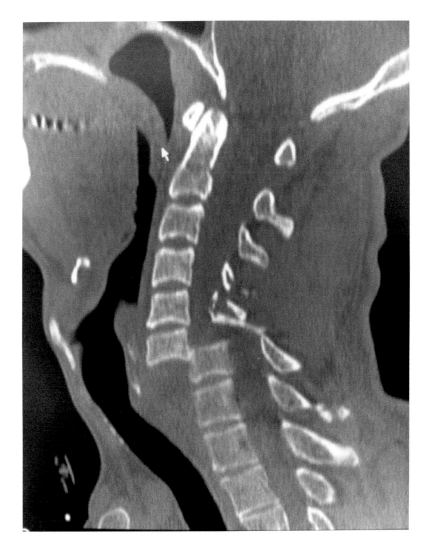

A 32-year-old woman is brought to the emergency department following a road traffic collision. She complains of neck pain and is immobilised in a cervical collar with blocks and on a spinal board. The initial ATLS assessment suggests that this is an isolated injury and there is no obvious neurologic deficit. She is imaged with CT and cuts of this study are shown here.

1. **Describe the initial investigation and management of this patient.**

   This CT image shows an anterolisthesis of the vertebral bodies of C6 on C7 of approximately 100% of the width of the vertebral body. This suggests a bilateral facet dislocation. Spinal precautions should be maintained and the neurologic status confirmed. I would discuss this patient with the local spinal surgery team and my initial management would be guided depending on their advice and local arrangements as the patient is likely to need specialist input and surgery.

   In general terms, for an awake and responsive patient able to understand and comply with instructions and without neurologic deficit, an attempt at closed reduction can be made using Gardner–Wells tongs and I would perform this in the operating theatre. An initial load of 10 lbs is applied and a lateral cervical spine radiograph is taken to identify any over-distraction, occult cervical spine fracture or occipitocervical instability. The weight is increased by 10–15 lbs every 15 minutes with repeat x-rays and assessments of the neurology until reduction is achieved. A slight extension moment can help to maintain the reduction once achieved. The weight is then reduced to 10–15 lbs and a rigid cervical collar applied. I would arrange a post-reduction MRI to help with surgical planning and would temporarily remove the tongs for this to be performed.

   If the patient develops abnormal neurology during the traction procedure I would stop and slowly release the traction continuing to monitor the patient to determine if the neurology normalises, remains static or is progressive. I would then immobilise the cervical spine and obtain an MRI.

   In situations where the patient is not awake or able to provide feedback during the procedure, reduction should be preceded by an MRI scan to exclude a posteriorly herniated disc.

2. **Following reduction of this injury, how would you proceed?**

   Bilateral facet dislocations are potentially associated with a significant posterior ligamentous injury and are likely to need definitive operative treatment. While awaiting this I would maintain rigid collar immobilisation and traction with the Gardner–Wells tongs and 10–15 lbs of weight. I would arrange post reduction radiographs to confirm the reduction, a post-reduction MRI to exclude disc herniation, spinal haematoma or other occult pathology and I would discuss this patient again with the local spinal service.

   I would choose an anterior cervical approach to allow a discectomy to be performed in the case of an extruded disc followed by a posterior cervical stabilisation with segmental screws. If the MRI shows no evidence of disc herniation then I would proceed directly to a posterior cervical stabilisation.

FURTHER READING

Lee JY, Nassr A, Eck JC, Vaccaro AR. Controversies in the treatment of cervical spine dislocations. *Spine J.* 2009 May;9(5):418–423. doi: 10.1016/j.spinee.2009.01.005. Epub 2009 Feb 23.

30

THORACOLUMBAR SPINE INJURY

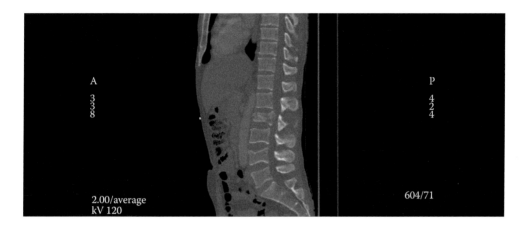

A 44-year-old man has jumped from the fifth floor of a building and has been brought to the emergency department. He is complaining of back pain and spinal precautions have been taken. This is an image from the CT taken in the emergency department.

1. **How would you investigate and manage this patient in the emergency department?**
   This patient should be treated along ATLS guidelines to ensure that life- and limb-threatening injuries are identified and treated appropriately. With respect to this specific injury, I would maintain spinal precautions and examine the patient carefully looking for any sign of neurological deficit.
   The CT shows a fracture at the level of L2. This is a burst fracture pattern with involvement of the anterior, middle and posterior columns. The CT image shows significant loss of vertebral height and retropulsion of fracture fragments and spinal canal compromise.

2. **What are the indications for surgery in this injury?**
   Fractures with associated neurological injury should be considered for surgery as should fractures where there is 30 degrees or more of kyphosis, compromise of the spinal canal by 50% or more and where there is progressive collapse into kyphosis or risk of this. I would also consider surgery in polytraumatised patients or where bracing is ineffective because of other injuries or body habitus. Loss of 50% of vertebral height or more suggests injury to the posterior ligamentous complex and resulting instability. Most other fractures can be treated in a thoracolumbar spinal orthosis (TLSO) to be worn whenever the patient is upright. If there is any doubt as to the stability of a fracture then I would arrange for an MRI to examine the integrity of the posterior ligamentous complex. I would check that bracing maintains satisfactory position with serial standing radiographs following application of the TLSO.
   These indications for surgery have been consolidated into an injury scoring system, the Thoracolumbar Injury Classification and Severity Score (TLICS), which incorporates injury morphology, posterior ligamentous complex integrity and

neurological status. A score of 4 is said to be the threshold at which operative management is considered.

3. **What surgical approach would you use for this fracture and which levels would you choose to stabilise?**

Surgery aims to decompress neural elements where required, reduce persisting spinal deformity, provide mechanical stability to spinal elements and allow bony healing.

Where decompression is required, I would achieve this through an anterior approach. For this patient who is neurologically intact I would choose a posterior approach to reduce residual kyphosis and achieve instrumented segmental fusion using pedicle screws. In this case, I would instrument one level above and two levels below the fracture level. In cases of very poor bone quality or where the vertebral body has lost 50% or more of its original height then short segment fusion would be more prone to failure and I would instrument two levels above and below the fracture.

4. **What do you understand about the terms *neurogenic shock* and *spinal shock*?**

Neurogenic shock results from disruption of the sympathetic pathways in the spinal cord with resultant uncontrolled peripheral vasodilation, a decrease in peripheral vascular resistance and a profound reduction in blood pressure. Depending on the level of spinal cord injury, there may also be a loss of sympathetic cardiac innervation with a resultant bradycardia. These features allow differentiation from hypovolaemic shock where the patient will appear peripherally shut down and tachycardic.

The term *spinal shock* refers to the complete loss of all neurological activity (motor, sensory, reflex and autonomic) below the level of spinal cord injury. Following a variable time period, from several days up to 6 weeks, spinal reflexes are expected to return and eventually become exaggerated as the syndrome of spasticity develops.

FURTHER READING

Wood KB, Buttermann GR, Phukan R, Harrod CC, Mehbod A, Shannon B, Bono CM, Harris MB. Operative compared with nonoperative treatment of a thoracolumbar burst fracture without neurological deficit: A prospective randomized study with follow-up at sixteen to twenty-two years. *J Bone Joint Surg Am.* 2015 Jan 7;97(1):3–9. doi: 10.2106/JBJS.N.00226.

31

PROXIMAL HUMERUS FRACTURE

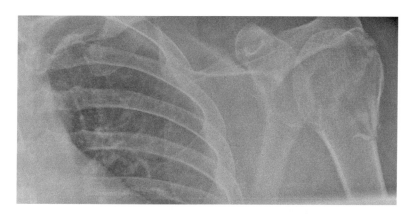

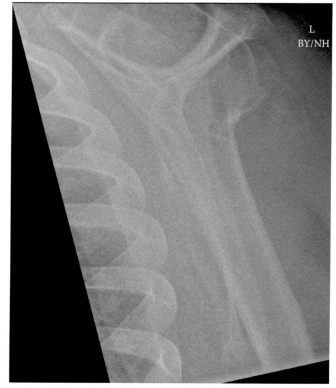

An 80-year-old woman attends the fracture clinic after stumbling and hitting her shoulder against a banister.

1. Describe these radiographs.

These are AP and axillary lateral views of the proximal humerus. They show a minimally displaced proximal humerus fracture.

2. How would you manage this patient?

I would make a careful clinical assessment of the patient and from the history and examination I would want to confirm that this is an isolated low-energy injury, the state of the soft tissues and any neurovascular deficit. I would make an assessment of the functional requirements of this patient. I would expect that this minimally displaced fracture pattern would be best treated non-operatively for this patient.

I would treat this patient in a collar and cuff and would follow-up with her in the fracture clinic. I would prescribe physiotherapy-supervised early active movement from the 3-week point post-injury.

3. What indications would make you consider operative intervention?

I would choose operative intervention for open fractures or where the skin is threatened or compromised, a vascular injury or a floating shoulder. Otherwise, surgery would be directed to obtain improved functional outcome. Fractures where surgery is likely to achieve this include head-splitting fractures, fractures with marked displacement which may predispose to mal- or non-union and especially where there is articular disruption.

FURTHER READING

Murray IR, Amin AK, White TO, Robinson CM. Proximal humeral fractures: Current concepts in classification, treatment and outcomes. *J Bone Joint Surg Br.* 2011 Jan;93(1):1–11. Review.

Torrens C, Corrales M, Vilà G, Santana F, Cáceres E. Functional and quality-of-life results of displaced and nondisplaced proximal humeral fractures treated conservatively. *J Orthop Trauma.* 2011 Oct;25(10):581–587.

32

PROXIMAL HUMERUS FRACTURE

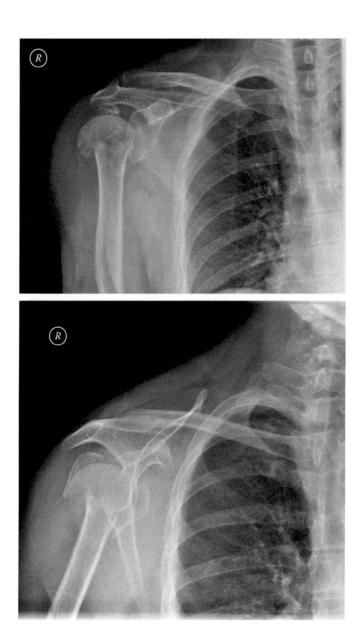

You are called to see a 55-year-old man in the emergency department. He has fallen 6 feet from a ladder. This is an isolated injury.

1. **Describe these radiographs.**
   These are AP and axillary lateral views of the proximal humerus. They show a displaced proximal humerus fracture.

2. How would you manage this isolated injury in this patient?

I would make a careful clinical assessment of the patient based on the history and examination. I would want to establish a number of key patient- and injury-related factors important for decision making. These include hand dominance, occupation and activities, functional demands and co-morbidities. Fracture-related factors include mechanism of injury, open fractures, associated neurovascular deficit, skin compromise and ipsilateral limb or shoulder girdle fractures.

This is an isolated injury but with obvious fracture displacement. For a relatively young patient with reasonable functional demands and expectations, I would recommend surgery in order to avoid potentially painful mal- or non-union and to obtain the best chance of a good functional outcome.

3. What surgery would you recommend and what would you tell the patient?

I would plan to fix this fracture using a proximal humerus locking plate through a deltopectoral approach.

I would tell the patient that surgery is generally safe and is likely to give him the best functional outcome and to avoid potentially painful mal- or non-union. There are a number of different techniques and while my preference and experience is to use a particular locked proximal humerus plate, there is little evidence to suggest that this is superior to other methods of fracture fixation. Despite this, there are risks inherent with any operation. Risks specific to this injury and operation include failure of fixation, neurovascular injury, shoulder stiffness, osteonecrosis and infection. These are rare and where avoided, the reported results are good. It is possible that for a patient with very low functional demands, non-operative treatment may allow healing with a functional result, but for a more active or physiologically younger patient, surgery does this more reliably although a multi-centre randomised trial (the PROFHER trial) did not find any difference in the outcomes of surgically and non-surgically treated patients after 2 years.

FURTHER READING

Murray IR, Amin AK, White TO, Robinson CM. Proximal humeral fractures: Current concepts in classification, treatment and outcomes. *J Bone Joint Surg Br.* 2011 Jan;93(1):1–11.

Rangan A, Handoll H, Brealey S, Jefferson L, Keding A, Martin BC, Goodchild L, Chuang LH, Hewitt C, Torgerson D, PROFHER Trial Collaborators. Surgical vs nonsurgical treatment of adults with displaced fractures of the proximal humerus: The PROFHER randomized clinical trial. *JAMA.* 2015 Mar 10;313(10):1037–1047. doi: 10.1001/jama .2015.1629.

Robinson CM, Amin AK, Godley KC, Murray IR, White TO. Modern perspectives of open reduction and plate fixation of proximal humerus fractures. *J Orthop Trauma.* 2011 Oct;25(10):618–629.

Torrens C, Corrales M, Vilà G, Santana F, Cáceres E. Functional and quality-of-life results of displaced and nondisplaced proximal humeral fractures treated conservatively. *J Orthop Trauma.* 2011 Oct;25(10):581–587.

33

GREATER TUBEROSITY FRACTURE

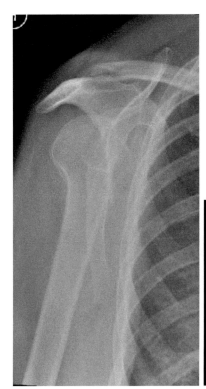
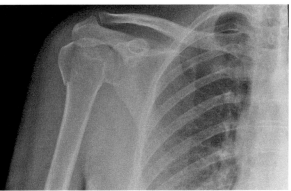

A 35-year-old woman fell from a ladder, injuring her right shoulder. These are her radiographs.

1. **What do the radiographs show?**
   This is an AP and 'Y' lateral view of the shoulder. It shows a fracture of the greater tuberosity which is undisplaced.

2. **How would you manage this patient?**
   I would take a careful history from this woman and perform a full examination. Assuming this is an isolated injury, I would look carefully for an associated undisplaced fracture of the surgical neck or proximal humerus. If there was any doubt then I would arrange a CT scan. The greater tuberosity fracture fragment may have a tendency to retract due to the pull of supraspinatus and infraspinatus. The CT would allow me to judge the true amount of displacement. Healing in a retracted position could result in impingement and defunctioning of the rotator cuff. Fracture fragment displacement greater than 5 mm is a relative indication for surgery.

   If the CT confirms the apparent injury of an undisplaced greater tuberosity fracture only then would I treat this patient in a sling for comfort and follow up clinically and radiographically at 1 week. I would allow her to start a programme of shoulder physiotherapy from the 3-week point, starting with active pendular movements and gentle passive range of movement.

If significant displacement is confirmed on CT or if subsequent displacement is noticed at follow-up then I would offer surgery. I would approach the fracture through a deltoid-splitting approach. For a large fracture fragment, as shown here, I would use 4 mm cannulated cancellous screws. Non-absorbable suture fixation would be an alternative should this not be possible.

3. What degree of displacement would make you consider operative fixation?
There is debate about this. I would consider operative fixation for a greater tuberosity fracture displaced by 5 mm or more or where the fracture fragment is in a position likely to cause impingement should it heal there.

FURTHER READING

DeBottis D, Anavian J, Green A. Surgical management of isolated greater tuberosity fractures of the proximal humerus. *Orthop Clin North Am.* 2014 Apr;45(2):207–218.

Janssen SJ, Hermanussen HH, Guitton TG, van den Bekerom MP, van Deurzen DF, Ring D. Greater tuberosity fractures: Does fracture assessment and treatment recommendation vary based on imaging modality? *Clin Orthop Relat Res.* 2016 May;474(5):1257–1265.

Rouleau DM, Mutch J, Laflamme GY. Surgical treatment of displaced greater tuberosity fractures of the humerus. *J Am Acad Orthop Surg.* 2016 Jan;24(1):46–56.

34

ANTERIOR SHOULDER DISLOCATION

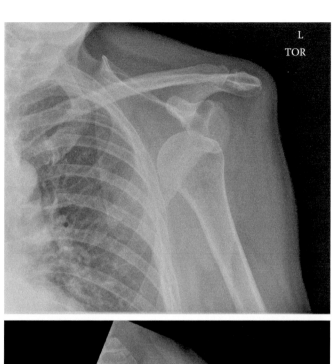

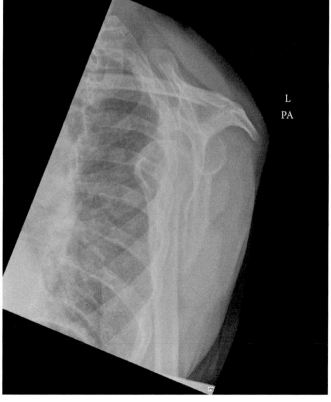

You are called to the emergency department to see a 60-year-old man who has fallen while running, injuring his shoulder. These are his radiographs.

1. **Describe these x-rays.**

   These are AP and modified axillary views of the shoulder, which show an anterior dislocation. There is no obvious sign of any associated fracture.

2. **How would you manage this patient in the emergency department?**

   I would undertake a full history and examination, confirming the mechanism and acute nature of the injury, hand dominance, occupation and activities and important co-morbidities. My examination would include a careful neurovascular assessment. This condition requires emergent care. If the patient is in pain I would administer analgesia and would plan to undertake closed reduction of the joint. In my unit, this is done in the emergency department under intravenous sedation. The sedation is administered by an anaesthetist or senior emergency department doctor who is able to manage the airway as required while I would perform the joint reduction with the assistance of a second doctor or nurse. For this, my preferred technique is to use gentle but sustained longitudinal traction with counter-traction provided by a second person using a sheet around the body. I would be prepared for the rare situation where it is not possible to achieve joint reduction in this way. In this situation, I would defer further intervention until the next day routine trauma operating list. I would arrange to take the patient to the operating theatre to attempt a closed reduction with a formal general anaesthetic and muscle relaxant with the potential for open reduction of the joint, should this be needed.

   Following joint reduction, I would confirm the position with further radiographs and would scrutinise these for signs of any new associated fracture. I would place the patient in a polysling to immobilise him for comfort and protection.

3. **When would you see this patient in the fracture clinic and how would you manage him?**

   The patient is discharged once safe and the effects of the anaesthetic or sedation have worn off. I would review him in the outpatient clinic at 1 week where I would take him out of the sling and repeat my examination, looking specifically to determine that the shoulder is still in joint, ensure there is no neurovascular deficit, to determine his range of movement and any sign of a rotator cuff tear. I would repeat AP and axillary lateral radiographs to confirm enlocation and to identify any fractures. If all is well, I would refer him to start physiotherapy for shoulder rehabilitation and early active movement. I would leave him in the care of the therapists unless there was a problem.

4. **Would your management change if the patient was an 18-year-old rugby player who sustained the injury in a tackle?**

   One of the problems after shoulder dislocation is recurrent instability. There is evidence to suggest that this risk is highest for young males. The dislocation involves a capsulolabral avulsion and in most cases, non-operative management and shoulder rehabilitation allow dynamic shoulder stabilisers to compensate for injured static stabilisers. A patient sustaining this injury in a contact sport may be at an increased risk for recurrent instability and I would have a careful discussion in the clinic about this. This is particularly relevant for young males. If the patient would consider the potential for early surgery or wish to continue contact sporting activities, I would investigate him with an MR arthrogram to look for any evidence of a Bankart lesion, significant glenoid injury or Hill–Sachs lesion. This would give me further information to have a considered discussion with the patient about the risk of recurrent instability.

5. **Do you know of any papers or evidence to support your views?**
   There is some work from Itoi to suggest that bracing in external rotation after a first-time anterior dislocation reduces the risk of recurrence. This is thought to work by approximating the Bankart lesion to the neck of the glenoid so that it heals in an anatomic location. Many patients find this position impractical however, and results have not been as successful in other hands.

   Hovelius undertook a prospective study over 10 years of non-operative treatment of first-time shoulder dislocators. He identified a high (48%) rate of recurrent instability over this time frame.

   Reviewing his results over 25 years, half of the young patients remained stable or became stable over time but he still identified that 34% of patients had recurrent instability or underwent surgery to address this.

   Robinson has studied the natural history of the anterior shoulder dislocations and identified that in a series of 252 patients, 55.7% had recurrent instability after 2 years. The risk of instability is greatest for young males for whom early surgical stabilisation should be considered.

FURTHER READING

Hovelius L, Augustini BG, Fredin H, Johansson O, Norlin R, Thorling J. Primary anterior dislocation of the shoulder in young patients. A ten-year prospective study. *J Bone Joint Surg Am.* 1996 Nov;78(11):1677–1684.

Hovelius L, Olofsson A, Sandström B, Augustini BG, Krantz L, Fredin H, Tillander B, Skoglund U, Salomonsson B, Nowak J, Sennerby U. Nonoperative treatment of primary anterior shoulder dislocation in patients forty years of age and younger. A prospective twenty-five-year follow-up. *J Bone Joint Surg Am.* 2008 May;90(5):945–952.

Itoi E, Hatakeyama Y, Sato T, Kido T, Minagawa H, Yamamoto N, Wakabayashi I, Nozaka K. Immobilization in external rotation after shoulder dislocation reduces the risk of recurrence. A randomized controlled trial. *J Bone Joint Surg Am.* 2007 Oct;89(10):2124–2131.

Robinson CM, Howes J, Murdoch H, Will E, Graham C. Functional outcome and risk of recurrent instability after primary traumatic anterior shoulder dislocation in young patients. *J Bone Joint Surg Am.* 2006 Nov;88(11):2326–2336.

35

POSTERIOR DISLOCATION OF SHOULDER

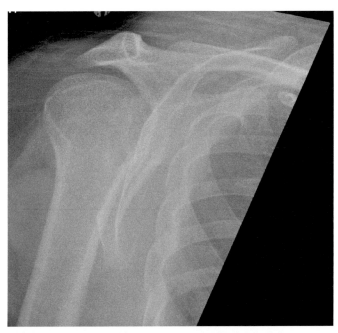

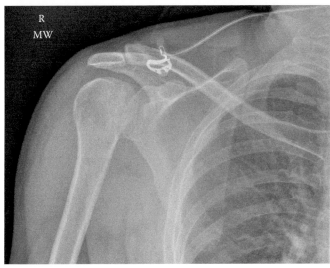

A 45-year-old man with epilepsy is brought to the emergency department following a seizure. He complains of right shoulder pain and these radiographs are taken.

1. **Describe the appearances in these radiographs.**

   These radiographs are an AP view of the shoulder and a scapular 'Y' view of the right shoulder. The images and the history are suggestive of a posterior dislocation of the shoulder. On these views, the humeral head has a 'lightbulb' appearance on the AP view due to its internally rotated position. The distance between the anterior rim of the glenoid and the humeral head is increased, there is a suggestion of a vertical line where there has been impaction on the humeral head from the posterior glenoid and the anterior glenoid appears empty.

2. **How would you investigate and assess this patient?**

   I would undertake a careful history and examination of this patient, trying to elucidate the age of the injury and any current neurovascular symptoms or deficit. I would expect to find the shoulder in fixed internal rotation or with very limited external rotation. I would be suspicious of an impaction fracture or defect in the humeral head from the posterior glenoid and a CT scan would help to define this. This would usually be in the anteromedial aspect of the humeral head, a reverse Hill–Sachs lesion, and so may contribute to ongoing posterior instability of the shoulder.

3. **How would you manage this patient?**

   In the acute situation, it may be possible to reduce this dislocation closed with good anaesthesia and formal muscle relaxation. I would have one careful attempt in the emergency department in the acute situation using sedation and with anaesthetic support. I would attempt reduction using a forward flexion, adduction and axial traction manouvre. I would attempt to unlock the humeral head from the posterior glenoid rim using direct lateral pressure on the humeral head followed by external rotation of the shoulder once unlocked. Should this fail then I would be prepared to take the patient to theatre for full general anaesthesia, muscle relaxation and the potential for an open reduction via a deltopectoral approach.

   I would be wary if there was any suggestion that this was a neglected injury older than 2 or 3 weeks, especially in an elderly osteoporotic patient. Chronic dislocations are more difficult to reduce closed and more likely to need open intervention. In addition, there is significant potential to make the situation worse in an osteoporotic patient where a soft humeral head impacted on the glenoid rim can be converted into a head-splitting fracture by overzealous manipulation.

   Once reduced, I would assess the stability of the shoulder through a range of movement, arrange further imaging with CT if not already done to assess any defect in the humeral head and place the patient in a sling.

4. **What reconstructive options might be available to this patient?**

   If the shoulder is stable then nothing further may be required. If the shoulder is unstable then surgical options might include transfer of the supraspinatus attachment/lesser tuberosity into the humeral head defect for a small to moderate-sized defect (up to 25% of the surface area). Instability with a larger defect could be addressed with an allograft fixation with or without a rotational osteotomy or joint arthroplasty surgery.

FURTHER READING

Cicak N. Posterior dislocation of the shoulder. *J Bone Joint Surg Br.* 2004 Apr;86(3):324–332. Review.

Robinson CM, Seah M, Akhtar MA. The epidemiology, risk of recurrence, and functional outcome after an acute traumatic posterior dislocation of the shoulder. *J Bone Joint Surg Am.* 2011 Sep 7;93(17):1605–1613.

Rouleau DM, Hebert-Davies J, Robinson CM. Acute traumatic posterior shoulder dislocation. *J Am Acad Orthop Surg.* 2014 Mar;22(3):145–152.

36

CLAVICLE FRACTURE

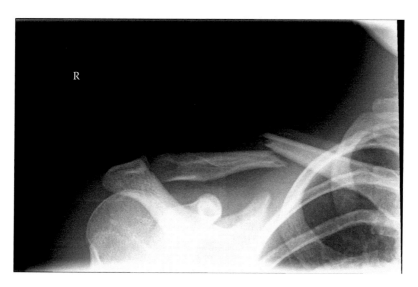

A 28-year-old woman presents to the emergency department after a fall from a horse. The emergency department doctor has diagnosed a clavicle fracture from this radiograph.

1. **How would you treat this injury in the emergency department?**

   I would take a careful history and examine the patient, looking for signs of any open wound, significant soft tissue contusion, degloving, threatened or tented skin and any associated injuries. I would look closely for any neurovascular injury. I would ensure that the patient had sufficient analgesia and would advise that they rest the upper limb in a polysling. I would review the radiograph for displacement, comminution and fracture pattern, and, if required, repeat this to ensure that I had a representative AP and tilted view (30-degree cephalad) to make this assessment.

2. **What advice would you give this patient about treatment options?**

   I would advise this patient that the vast majority of these fractures will heal satisfactorily. For a closed fracture pattern such as this in a fit and healthy patient I would advise the use of a simple sling and analgesia for comfort and that this can be discontinued once pain allows.

   I would warn the patient that there is a risk that the fracture may not unite and this is of the order of 15% or so. I would advise that surgery can reduce this risk of non-union to approximately 3% and may allow an earlier return to work or function, but surgery does introduce other risks such as infection, injury to nerves and blood vessels, painful or prominent metalwork, the need for further surgery, anaesthetic risk, and there will be a scar, which may be sensitive.

3. **What would be your indications for operative treatment of a middle third clavicle fracture?**

Indications for operative treatment would include open fractures, threatened skin, vascular injury, scapulothoracic dissociation and neurologic deficit, especially where this is progressive.

Fracture comminution, representing a high-energy injury and a lack of cortical contact, are both features that have been shown to be predictive for non-union and would be relative indications for operative treatment.

Other relative indications would include a polytraumatised patient, a floating shoulder or where there is an ipsilateral upper limb injury.

FURTHER READING

Altamimi SA, McKee MD, Canadian Orthopaedic Trauma Society. Nonoperative treatment compared with plate fixation of displaced midshaft clavicular fractures. Surgical technique. *J Bone Joint Surg Am*. 2008 Mar;90 Suppl 2 Pt 1:1–8.

McKee RC, Whelan DB, Schemitsch EH, McKee MD. Operative versus nonoperative care of displaced midshaft clavicular fractures: A meta-analysis of randomized clinical trials. *J Bone Joint Surg Am*. 2012 Apr 18;94(8):675–684. Review.

Naimark M, Dufka FL, Han R, Sing DC, Toogood P, Ma CB, Zhang AL, Feeley BT. Plate fixation of midshaft clavicular fractures: Patient-reported outcomes and hardware-related complications. *J Shoulder Elbow Surg*. 2016 May;25(5):739–746.

Robinson CM, Goudie EB, Murray IR, Jenkins PJ, Ahktar MA, Read EO, Foster CJ, Clark K, Brooksbank AJ, Arthur A, Crowther MA, Packham I, Chesser TJ. Open reduction and plate fixation versus nonoperative treatment for displaced midshaft clavicular fractures: A multi-center, randomized, controlled trial. *J Bone Joint Surg Am*. 2013 Sep 4;95(17):1576–1584.

37

ACROMIOCLAVICULAR JOINT INJURY

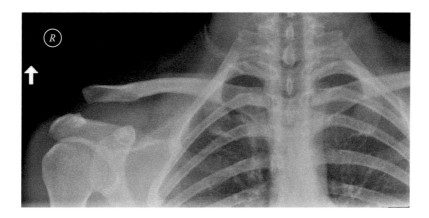

This is a radiograph of a patient brought to the emergency department after being knocked off his bicycle in a low-velocity road traffic accident. He complained of pain and deformity around the shoulder.

1. **Describe the appearances in this radiograph.**

   This is a plain radiograph of the left shoulder and the obvious abnormality is an increase in the acromioclavicular joint space and malalignment of the distal clavicle with the acromion representing a dislocation of the acromioclavicular joint.

2. **In your clinical assessment of this patient, what associated injuries might you specifically look for?**

   Having completed an assessment of the patient along ATLS guidelines and established that this is truly an isolated injury I would pay close attention to the condition of the soft tissues, looking for signs of any open wound and any suggestion that the overlying skin may be degloved, puckered or under tension. I would conduct a careful neurovascular assessment to identify any deficit. These injuries can be associated with brachial plexus injuries, although these are not common. I would look carefully for clinical or radiographic signs of associated fractures of the clavicle, acromion, coracoid or scapula.

3. **Assuming that this is an isolated injury, how would you manage this patient definitively?**

   There is demonstrable widening of the acromioclavicular joint space with the distal clavicle shown to lie superior to the superior border of the acromion and a marked increase in the coraco-clavicular distance. In the Rockwood system of classification this is a type V injury and I would offer surgery. Options include surgical coraco-clavicular ligament repair, LARS reconstruction, clavicle hook plate fixation or a modified Weaver–Dunn procedure. My preference would be to perform a modified Weaver–Dunn procedure through a bra-strap incision. The distal end of the clavicle is excised before reducing the clavicle into position and transferring the coracoacromial ligament to the lateral end of the clavicle. The reconstruction is augmented with three double strands of number 2 PDS sutures placed around the clavicle and under the coracoid and tied off anteriorly. I would advise the use of a sling postoperatively for 3 weeks but allow pendulum exercises. I would allow the patient to progress their therapy 3 weeks after reconstruction.

FURTHER READING

Beitzel K, Cote MP, Apostolakos J, Solovyova O, Judson CH, Ziegler CG, Edgar CM, Imhoff AB, Arciero RA, Mazzocca AD. Current concepts in the treatment of acromioclavicular joint dislocations. *Arthroscopy.* 2013 Feb;29(2):387–397.

Bradley JP, Elkousy H. Decision making: Operative versus nonoperative treatment of acromioclavicular joint injuries. *Clin Sports Med.* 2003 Apr;22(2):277–290.

38

MIDSHAFT HUMERUS FRACTURE

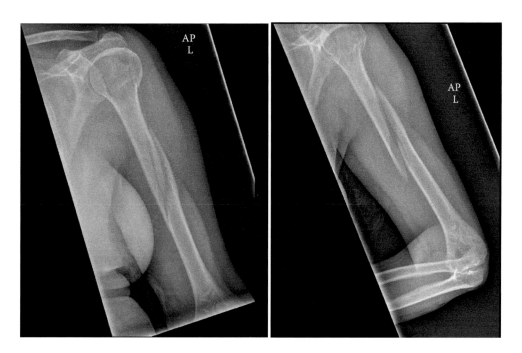

A 46-year-old man fell from a ladder, injuring his left non-dominant arm. This is an isolated injury and these are his radiographs from the emergency department.

1. **What do the radiographs show and how would you manage this patient?**
   These are plain radiographs of the left humerus. They show a displaced midshaft diaphyseal fracture.

   I would take a careful history from the patient and perform a full circumferential examination of the limb, looking for any sign of any open wound, significant soft tissue injury or ipsilateral fracture. I would perform an examination of the peripheral neurology and vascular status of the limb. Assuming that this is normal, I would place the limb in a hanging U-slab and repeat the radiographs and neurovascular assessment. If this was satisfactory I would plan to treat the patient with early functional bracing.

2. **What degree of residual displacement or deformity would you consider to be acceptable for non-operative treatment?**
   I would accept 20 degrees of angulation in the sagittal plane and 30 degrees of angulation in the coronal plane.

3. **You reassess the neurology and vascular status following application of a plaster cast and you note that the patient has developed altered sensation in the distribution of the radial nerve and a wrist drop. He is complaining of increased pain. How would you proceed?**

   The patient has developed radial nerve symptoms since the plaster cast was applied. I would remove the plaster cast and reassess the patient. If these symptoms persist then this would be a relative indication for surgical treatment although some surgeons might treat this more expectantly. Having had normal radial nerve function on presentation and a clear deterioration after manipulation or plaster cast application, I would plan to explore the nerve and internally fix the fracture on the next available routine trauma list. In the meantime I would ensure that the patient has adequate analgesia and is comfortable either in a collar and cuff or sling.

4. **What would be your indications for operative treatment for a midshaft diaphyseal humerus fracture?**

   Indications for operative treatment include open fractures, an associated vascular injury, ipsilateral fractures, floating shoulder or elbow, bilateral humerus fractures, polytrauma, failure to obtain and maintain an acceptable closed reduction, pathologic fractures, neurologic or brachial plexus injuries, intra-articular fracture or extension and unfavourable body habitus, particularly in ladies with large breasts, which might act as a fulcrum at the fracture site.

5. **What would you tell the patient about the risks and benefits of operative versus non-operative treatment?**

   Both treatment options have similar times to union and rates of union. Rates of non-union for midshaft diaphyseal fractures treated with functional bracing are 2–10% but slightly higher for more proximal or long oblique fracture patterns. Compression plating has been found to have a non-union rate around 5–10%. Operative treatment does expose the patient to the risks of iatrogenic nerve or vessel injury and infection but will allow earlier movement of the arm once stabilised. Functional bracing avoids the risks of surgery but may be associated with a longer duration of initial discomfort and pain while the fracture fragments are mobile and there is a higher risk of mal-union, although this may not be of any consequence.

6. **How does the Sarmiento functional brace work?**

   The brace is applied once pain allows and may need to be adjusted once initial swelling settles. The brace is made up of overlapping synthetic plastic shells lined with soft foam and fitted to the arm. The shells are contoured to fit the biceps and triceps. They are held with Velcro straps and encircle the arm, applying a compressive force to the soft tissues controlling and splinting the humeral fracture segments. Gravity also assists the realignment of fracture segments. Functional bracing of these midshaft fractures allows for some movement of the elbow and shoulder over the course of treatment, reducing unnecessary joint stiffness.

FURTHER READING

Klenerman L. Fractures of the shaft of the humerus. *J Bone Joint Surg Br.* 1966 Feb;48(1):105–111.

Sarmiento A, Zagorski JB, Zych GA, Latta LL, Capps CA. Functional bracing for the treatment of fractures of the humeral diaphysis. *J Bone Joint Surg Am.* 2000 Apr;82(4):478–486.

Shao YC, Harwood P, Grotz MR, Limb D, Giannoudis PV. Radial nerve palsy associated with fractures of the shaft of the humerus: A systematic review. *J Bone Joint Surg Br.* 2005 Dec;87(12):1647–1652.

39

HOLSTEIN–LEWIS FRACTURE

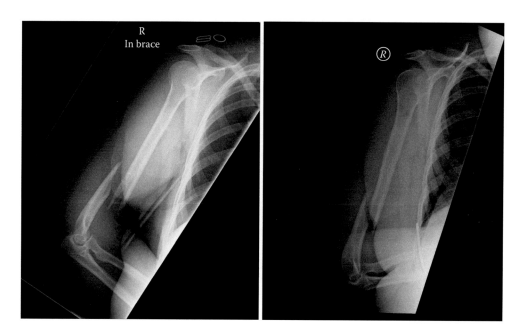

A 32-year-old man is admitted with an injury to his right arm. He has a dense radial nerve palsy. He tells you that this happened while arm wrestling.

1. Describe these radiographs.

These are an AP radiograph of the right humerus and a lateral radiograph of the distal humerus and elbow. These show a displaced fracture in the distal third of the humerus.

2. Do you anticipate any potential problems with this fracture pattern?

This particular fracture pattern is often referred to as a Holstein–Lewis fracture. The fracture is at the distal third of the humerus in close proximity to the radial nerve as it passes posteriorly and around the radial aspect of the humerus and through the lateral intermuscular septum where it is in close contact with bone. The radial nerve may become injured through laceration, contusion or stretch at the time of injury and at surgery it has also been found entrapped between displaced fracture fragments.

There is some debate about how this fracture type should be ideally managed. The evidence shows that the vast majority of nerve injuries involve a neurapraxia and resolve over 3–6 months with non-operative treatment. Many surgeons believe that these distal fractures are difficult to manage with splints or braces although there are several reported series with good results. This fracture pattern is often considered a relative indication for surgery because of the relatively more common association with radial nerve injury and a perceived risk of non-union or elbow stiffness associated with brace or cast treatment although this is not supported by the literature.

3. **If this is an isolated closed injury, how would you assess and advise this patient?**
I would undertake a full history and examination of the patient, paying particular attention to the condition of the soft tissues, any open injuries and the neurological and vascular status of the patient.

I would discuss the benefits of operative and non-operative treatment with the patient and if amenable, I would apply a coaptation splint and repeat the radiographs to assess the reduction. If the fracture is reduced and held in an acceptable position then functional bracing would be my preferred treatment. I would advise that most nerve injuries recover fully over time and I would expect to see clinical signs of improvement within 6–8 weeks, with full recovery by 3–6 months. I would obtain an EMG study after 4 weeks to assess radial nerve recovery.

If an acceptable reduction cannot be achieved, then I would advise operative treatment with exploration of the nerve and fracture fixation. I would be prepared to undertake nerve repair or grafting with the assistance of a plastic surgery colleague.

4. **If you agree with the patient to proceed with surgical management, what procedure would you choose to undertake? Do you anticipate any potential problems and what surgical approach would you use?**
I would choose to treat this injury surgically with open exploration of the radial nerve and I would recruit the support of a plastic surgery colleague in case I should find that nerve repair is necessary at the time of surgery. My preference for fracture fixation would be compression plating. This is a distal fracture and so there is limited space for screw fixation in the distal fragment. I would use a posterior surgical approach as this offers good access with a flat surface for plate fixation and good visualisation of the nerve. I would identify the nerve on the posterior surface of the humerus above the medial head of the triceps and I would explore it distally to and beyond the fracture to identify and address any nerve injury. I would reduce and plate the fracture in compression mode using a narrow 4.5 mm LC-DC plate for this.

Following fracture fixation, if the nerve is simply contused then I would ensure that it is free of tension and not directly on the plate surface. If the nerve is seen to be lacerated or if there is a segmental injury, then options for treatment would include direct nerve repair, nerve grafting or late tendon transfers if initial treatment fails. I would consider these with the help of my plastic surgery colleague. I would record the final condition and position of the nerve carefully in the operative note so as to make any later surgical approach safer.

I would apply simple soft dressings and allow early movement unless a nerve repair or graft has been performed, as that would need to be protected with a short period of splintage in a plaster backslab.

FURTHER READING

Ekholm R, Ponzer S, Törnkvist H, Adami J, Tidermark J. The Holstein-Lewis humeral shaft fracture: Aspects of radial nerve injury, primary treatment, and outcome. *J Orthop Trauma*. 2008 Nov–Dec;22(10):693–697.

40

DISTAL HUMERUS FRACTURE

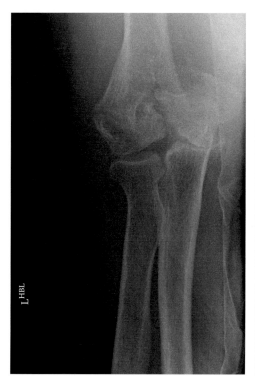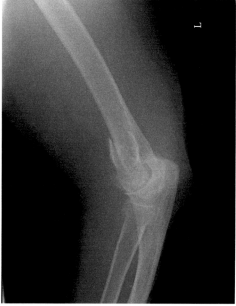

A 66-year-old man is admitted to the orthopaedic unit after a fall in which he injured his elbow. This is an isolated injury.

1. **Describe these radiographs.**

   These are AP and lateral radiographs of the left elbow showing a displaced, intra-articular and comminuted fracture of the distal humerus.

2. **Assuming that this is an isolated closed injury in a patient who is medically fit and well with high-functional demands, how would you plan to treat this injury?**

   This is an intra-articular injury. My preference for an active patient with high functional demands would be for open reduction and internal fixation using a double plating technique in order to achieve satisfactory fracture stability so that early movement can be instituted. I would review the history and undertake a full examination, including an assessment of the soft tissues and neurovascular status. Further imaging, particularly CT imaging, might give me further information regarding the number of fragments, the degree of comminution and guide my preoperative planning.

3. **What surgical approach would you use? Which implants would you use and where would you place them?**

I would use a posterior surgical approach, identifying the ulnar nerve and decompressing or transposing it first as appropriate before performing a chevron olecranon osteotomy. The tip of the osteotomy should be distally directed in order to avoid splitting the proximal fragment and should be performed through the 'bare area' of the olecranon. I would pre-drill the osteotomy to allow for fixation at the end of the procedure with a 6.5 mm cannulated cancellous screw and washer. This approach offers improved visibility and access to the distal fracture fragments.

I would use a double plating technique and would choose anatomic pre-contoured distal humerus locking plates placed along the medial column and the lateral columns using the parallel plating technique as described by O'Driscoll and I would aim to maximise fixation in the distal fragment.

4. **What problems do you anticipate with your treatment choice?**

There are several potential problems.

This is a very low and comminuted distal humerus fracture in what appears to be radiographically osteopenic bone. It may not be technically possible to fix this fracture as it is a very small distal fragment which is already comminuted and it may prove difficult to get good purchase distally. This may predispose to failure of fixation, delayed or non-union as movement occurs preferentially at the fracture site rather than at the elbow joint. In addition, surgery around the elbow is often associated with heterotopic ossification as well as post-traumatic or post-surgical stiffness.

5. **Are there any other options available if you are unable to fix this fracture?**

Alternative treatment options might include non-operative treatment, particularly for the frail or low-demand patient, known as the 'bag of bones' treatment method. Alternatively, total elbow arthroplasty or even distal humerus hemiarthroplasty might be used. If total elbow arthroplasty is under consideration then an olecranon osteotomy should not be used. In this situation, I would approach the fracture using a para-tricipital approach creating operative windows on either side of the triceps in order to visualise the fracture directly.

6. **Can you tell me about any problems with the use of total elbow replacement (TEA) for distal humerus fractures?**

When total elbow replacement is used for trauma it is usually because the fracture is too comminuted to satisfactorily fix. This level of injury may mean that the medial and lateral columns of the distal humerus are unreconstructable and the collateral ligaments may also be badly injured. In order to obtain a stable elbow replacement, it is often necessary to use a linked implant, which may contribute to a higher rate of bearing surface wear and implant loosening. A lifting restriction (commonly 5 kg) is usually imposed for these patients to try to limit this. Also, younger and more active patients treated with TEA for trauma have poorer satisfaction scores, more complications and a higher rates of loosening than low-demand patients.

Even in low-demand patients, an elbow replacement is at risk of subsequent prosthetic infection, periprosthetic fracture, loosening and wear – all of which may require further (difficult) surgery.

FURTHER READING

Aitken SA, Jenkins PJ, Rymaszewski L. Revisiting the 'bag of bones': Functional outcome after the conservative management of a fracture of the distal humerus. *Bone Joint J.* 2015 Aug;97-B(8):1132–1138.

McKee MD, Veillette CJ, Hall JA, Schemitsch EH, Wild LM, McCormack R, Perey B, Goetz T, Zomar M, Moon K, Mandel S, Petit S, Guy P, Leung I. A multicenter, prospective, randomized, controlled trial of open reduction – Internal fixation versus total elbow-arthroplasty for displaced intra-articular distal humeral fractures in elderly patients. *J Shoulder Elbow Surg.* 2009 Jan–Feb;18(1):3–12.

Nauth A, McKee MD, Ristevski B, Hall J, Schemitsch EH. Distal humeral fractures in adults. *J Bone Joint Surg Am.* 2011 Apr 6;93(7):686–700. doi: 10.2106/JBJS.J.00845.

Prasad N, Ali A, Stanley D. Total elbow arthroplasty for non-rheumatoid patients with a fracture of the distal humerus: A minimum ten-year follow-up. *Bone Joint J.* 2016 Mar;98-B(3):381–386.

Sanchez-Sotelo J, Torchia ME, O'Driscoll SW. Complex distal humeral fractures: Internal Internal fixation with a principle-based parallel-plate technique. *J Bone Joint Surg Am.* 2007 May;89(5):961–969.

41

ELBOW DISLOCATION

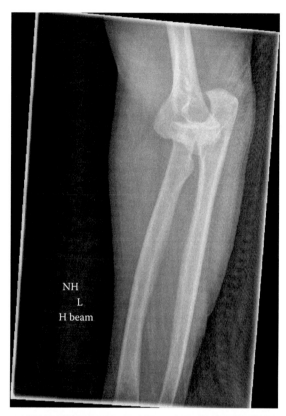

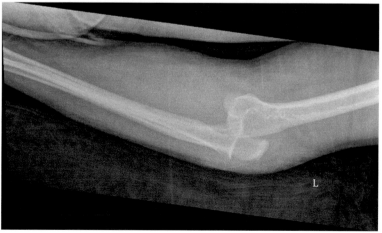

A 22-year-old man has injured his left arm in a rugby tackle. He is seen in the emergency department. These are his radiographs.

1. **What do these radiographs show and how would you manage this patient?**

   This are plain radiographs of the elbow in a skeletally mature individual and it shows a posterior dislocation of the elbow.

   Having completed my clinical assessment and documented the neurovascular status of the patient, I would plan to reduce the elbow dislocation. I would usually perform this under sedation in the emergency department. I would reduce the elbow by flexing it to 30 degrees in supination to unlock the olecranon from the olecranon fossa, applying longitudinal traction and gently levering or pushing the olecranon over the distal humerus. Occasionally this cannot be achieved under sedation, and in this situation, I would arrange to perform this in the operating theatre under general anaesthesia.

   Having reduced the elbow, I would take it through a gentle range of movement to confirm that a congruent reduction has been obtained and can be maintained. I would then place the patient in an above elbow backslab. Obvious gross instability or failure to achieve a congruent reduction may require further intervention, possibly open reduction, ligament repair or external fixation. I would confirm reduction with further x-rays in plaster and would review the patient in the fracture clinic at 1 week. At that time, I would remove the backslab before repeating my examination and taking further x-rays. I would plan to mobilise the patient actively from this time barring unexpected complications.

   Where it is not possible to obtain a closed reduction of the elbow, an open reduction is required. I would perform this in the operating theatre using a tourniquet and accessing the elbow through Kocher's approach. Failure to achieve reduction may be because of interposed soft tissues, bony impaction or buttonholing of the radial head through the capsule.

2. **What structures do you think might be damaged in this injury?**

   The pathoanatomy of elbow dislocations has been described by O'Driscoll. He described a ring of instability where progressive instability is caused by sequential tearing of the soft tissues around the elbow. Typically, the patient falls on or axially loads the supinated forearm. The first structure to tear is the lateral collateral ligament (LCL), followed by the anterior capsule before the medial collateral ligament (MCL) is torn. For the elbow to be dislocated in this way, I would expect the lateral collateral ligament and the anterior capsule to be injured. The medial collateral ligament may also be injured. The lateral ulnar part of the LCL and the anterior bundle of the MCL are the more important components of the collateral ligaments for stability. Gross instability may result if the common flexor or extensor origins are avulsed.

3. **Having reduced the elbow and confirmed on x-ray that it goes back into the joint, you are unable to maintain this position because the elbow is grossly unstable. How would you manage this?**

   In this situation, further management in the emergency department is inappropriate. I would take the patient to theatre where I would attempt to reduce and immobilise the elbow in an above elbow backslab. If this failed I would explore the lateral side of the elbow in order to identify any tears in the LCL or common extensor origin and to repair these using suture anchors/sutures. If the elbow remained unstable, I would address the medial side of the elbow, looking for tears to the MCL and the common flexor origin, approaching it through the bed of the ulnar nerve. I would repair this with a heavy Orthocord® #2 suture. If the elbow remained unstable after this, I would apply an external fixator across the elbow to hold it in joint.

FURTHER READING

Anakwe RE, Middleton SD, Jenkins PJ, McQueen MM, Court-Brown CM. Patient-reported outcomes after simple dislocation of the elbow. *J Bone Joint Surg Am.* 2011 Jul 6;93(13):1220–1226.

O'Driscoll SW, Morrey BF, Korinek S, An KN. Elbow subluxation and dislocation. A spectrum of instability. *Clin Orthop Relat Res.* 1992 Jul;(280):186–197.

42

TERRIBLE TRIAD INJURY

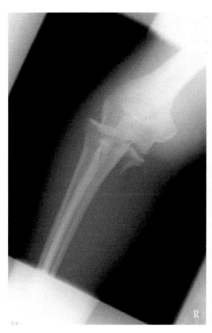 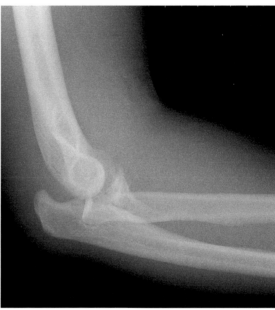

A 29-year-old man fell from a horse, injuring his right dominant elbow. He is seen in the fracture clinic and these are his radiographs from the emergency department.

1. **Describe the appearances of these radiographs and what structures you would expect to be injured.**

   These radiographs show a dislocation of the elbow associated with a displaced and comminuted fracture of the radial head. There is also a fracture of the coronoid. This combination is often referred to as a *terrible triad injury* and represents a high-energy injury. I would expect a degree of injury to the soft tissue stabilisers of the elbow. I would expect the lateral collateral ligament of the elbow to be injured as well as the anterior capsule of the elbow joint in association with the coronoid fracture. It is also possible that there could be a medial collateral ligament injury.

2. **What treatment would you advise for this injury?**

   This is an inherently unstable injury and I would advise operative treatment. I would specifically aim to restore ulnohumeral joint stability by reducing the dislocation and repairing the coronoid fracture. A preoperative CT scan would be helpful if this can be performed urgently. If the coronoid fragment is too small to fix then I would perform a suture repair of the anterior capsule to the proximal ulna. I would replace the radial head and repair the lateral collateral ligament. I would reassess the joint stability and fracture fixation. If this is satisfactory, as is usually the case, nothing further would be required. I would rest the elbow in an above elbow backslab for 2 weeks to protect the wound. If, following fixation, there was still residual instability I would consider a separate repair of the medial collateral ligament if examination suggested an injury here also. Otherwise I would consider augmenting the fixation by applying an external fixator across the elbow. CT imaging can be helpful in determining the degree of comminution, where fracture fragments have originated from and their degree of displacement, and I would request this preoperatively.

3. Describe your planned operative sequence for fixation and repair.
I would position the patient in the lateral position right side uppermost and with the arm across a bolster. I would ensure that preoperative antibiotics were administered and I would use a narrow sterile tourniquet. I would use the utility posterior approach to the elbow, raising thick flaps.

I would identify, decompress and protect the ulnar nerve in situ. I would identify any traumatic rent in the lateral structures and use this to develop access to the elbow, but if there is no clear soft tissue defect to access then I would use Kocher's interval between anconeus and extensor carpi ulnaris. I would excise the radial head fragments first, which would give me access to the coronoid and anterior capsule. Depending on coronoid fragment size I would reduce and fix the coronoid fracture with a single screw or I would suture the anterior capsule down to the coronoid footprint using suture anchors. Fractures to the anteromedial facet of the coronoid are less reliably secured using these methods and where this fracture type is identified in advance, I would approach the fracture fragment via a medial approach through the bed of the ulnar nerve. This would provide access to allow me to apply a buttress plate to the anteromedial surface of the coronoid.

I would then prepare and place a radial head replacement, taking care not to 'overstuff' the joint. I would confirm appropriate sizing of the radial head implant using trial implants radiographically and under direct vision: The ulnohumeral joint should be even radiographically; lateral gapping suggests an overstuffed joint. Under direct vision, the diameter of the implant should be matched to the size of the resected fragments and the prosthesis should sit so that it articulates with the radial notch and capitellum. Gapping of the coronoid away from the trochlea suggests overstuffing.

I would then confirm reduction of the ulnohumeral joint and perform a closure in layers including a repair of the lateral collateral ligament using a suture anchor.

FURTHER READING

Chen NC, Ring D. Terrible triad injuries of the elbow. *J Hand Surg Am.* 2015 Nov;40(11): 2297–2303.

Mathew PK, Athwal GS, King GJ. Terrible triad injury of the elbow: Current concepts. *J Am Acad Orthop Surg.* 2009 Mar;17(3):137–151.

43

RADIAL HEAD FRACTURE

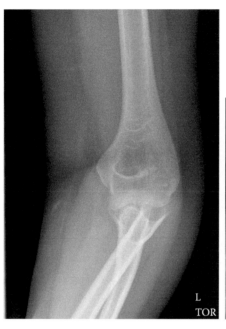
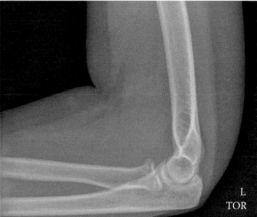

A 32-year-old man fell while rollerblading, injuring his left dominant elbow. He complained of pain and a reduced range of movement. These are the emergency department radiographs, which shows an isolated injury.

1. **How would you manage this patient?**
   This shows a minimally displaced fracture of the radial head. I would complete the history and a full examination of the patient, confirming that this is a closed injury and that there is no neurovascular deficit. I would ensure that the patient has adequate analgesia and would carefully try to assess the range of movement, accepting that this may be limited due to pain. I do not routinely aspirate the joint for haematoma as some surgeons might but I would place the patient in a collar and cuff and advise analgesia, early movement and physiotherapy. I would review the patient in the fracture clinic at the 2-week point to reassess them to ensure that their pain was settling, the range of movement was improving, there was no clear mechanical block to forearm rotation and there had not been any radiographic fracture displacement.

2. **What would your indications for surgery be?**
   I would consider surgery where a radial head fracture was associated with more complex fracture dislocations of the elbow where joint stability is compromised. I would also consider surgery for isolated fractures of the radial head which are open

injuries, where there is a mechanical block to movement or for displaced fractures where I anticipate that healing of the displaced fracture fragments in situ will result in impingement or subsequent loss of motion.

3. **How would you decide between fixation and replacement for comminuted fracture types?**

There is good evidence that where surgery is selected, open reduction and internal fixation are best reserved for non-comminuted fractures where there are three or fewer fracture fragments. Attempted fixation of more comminuted fractures is more often prone to failure of fixation and non-union. For more comminuted fracture patterns where the fracture is not fixable and where elbow stability may be compromised, radial head replacement may be more reliable. In addition, for isolated fractures of the radial head, there is still a place for radial head resection in non-repairable fractures where a careful assessment shows that the remaining stabilisers of the elbow joint are intact. In practice, non-repairable fracture patterns are often associated with higher-energy injuries, which have been shown to have a higher associated rate of ligamentous and other bony injuries and which need to be carefully excluded.

FURTHER READING

Duckworth AD, McQueen MM, Ring D. Fractures of the radial head. *Bone Joint J.* 2013 Feb;95-B(2):151–159.

Ring D, Quintero J, Jupiter JB. Open reduction and internal fixation of fractures of the radial head. *J Bone Joint Surg Am.* 2002 Oct;84-A(10):1811–1815.

44

OLECRANON FRACTURE

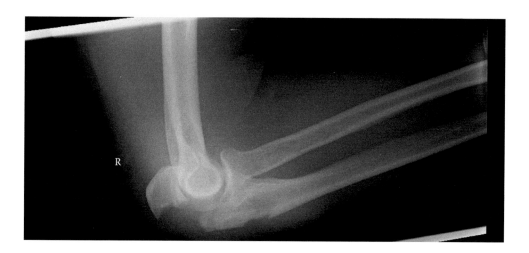

This is the radiograph of the elbow of a 40-year-old man who fell off his bicycle.

1. **What does the radiograph show and how would you manage this patient?**

   This is an AP and lateral radiograph of the right elbow. It shows a comminuted and displaced fracture of the olecranon.

   I would take a full history from this patient and perform a careful examination, looking particularly for evidence of any open wounds, significant soft tissue injury or any neurovascular deficit. I would ensure that the patient had adequate analgesia and I would apply an above elbow backslab to splint the limb. My advice would be that this injury should be treated definitively with surgery and I would choose to treat this patient with plate fixation.

2. **How would you choose between tension band wire fixation and plate fixation for an olecranon fracture?**

   My preference would be to use tension band wire fixation for simple pattern fractures at the level of the trochlear notch and proximally. For more complicated fracture patterns, fracture dislocations, injuries where the joint is subluxed or for comminuted fractures I would prefer plate fixation.

3. **Can you explain the principle that tension band fixation is based on?**

   A dorsally applied tension band converts the normally distractive (tensile) force of the triceps into a compressive force at the fracture site. The principle relies on bony contact at the volar cortex and so it is not suitable for fractures with significant comminution, which are better treated with plating.

4. Would you consider an alternative treatment for a frail 90-year-old woman with low-functional demands and significant co-morbidities and anaesthetic risks?
There is emerging evidence that non-operative treatment produces satisfactory functional outcomes for elderly patients with low functional demands even with displaced fractures of the olecranon. Patients are treated with pain relief, a short period of splintage and early mobilisation.

FURTHER READING

Das AK, Jariwala A, Watts AC. Suture repair of simple transverse olecranon fractures and chevron olecranon osteotomy. *Tech Hand Up Extrem Surg.* 2016 Mar;20(1):1–5.

Duckworth AD, Bugler KE, Clement ND, Court-Brown CM, McQueen MM. Nonoperative management of displaced olecranon fractures in low-demand elderly patients. *J Bone Joint Surg Am.* 2014 Jan 1;96(1):67–72.

Veillette CJ, Steinmann SP. Olecranon fractures. *Orthop Clin North Am.* 2008 Apr;39(2):229–236.

45

MONTEGGIA FRACTURE

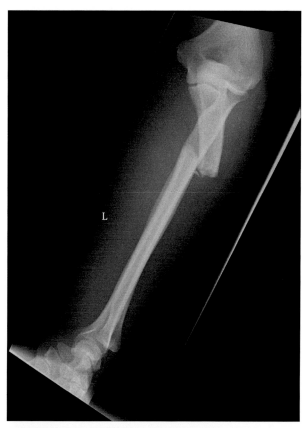

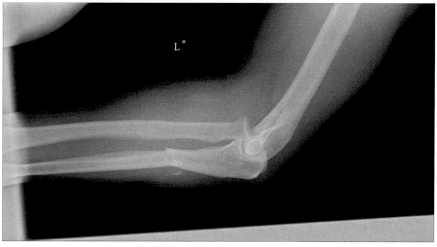

1. **Describe the appearances shown in these radiographs.**

   These are AP and lateral radiographs of the elbow that show a fracture of the proximal ulna and a dislocation of the radial head, referred to as a *Monteggia fracture dislocation*. The radial head appears to be dislocated anteriorly in this case.

2. **How would you choose to manage this injury?**

   As always, I would take a full history from and examine this patient. I would pay particular attention to identify any neurologic or vascular deficit. Having reviewed the patient and the radiographs I would plan to treat this operatively with reduction of the radiocapitellar joint and plate fixation of the ulna. I would position the patient in a lateral position, injured side uppermost and hang the arm over a bar to allow easy access to the dorsal surface. I would use a dorsal approach to the ulna, reduce the fracture and apply a 3.5 mm LC-DC plate to the ulna. I would apply the plate to the dorsal surface of the ulna. I would perform the surgery with image intensification to confirm the reduction. I would place the patient in an above elbow backslab postoperatively for a period of 2 weeks.

3. **Having reduced and fixed the ulna with plate fixation, you find that the radial head is still dislocated and is irreducible. How would you proceed?**

   I would screen the elbow dynamically using the image intensifier to confirm this. I would then examine my fixation of the ulna. Malreduction of the ulna is the most common cause for a failure to reduce the radiocapitellar joint. If the ulnar fixation looks satisfactory then I would consider whether there may be a soft tissue problem. The radial head may have buttonholed through a portion of anconeus, the capsule or have a portion of the annular ligament interposed in the joint. I would approach this through a separate Kocher's incision in order to perform an open reduction. In order to achieve reduction it may be necessary to remove all or part of the ulnar fixation.

FURTHER READING

Ring D. Monteggia fractures. *Orthop Clin North Am.* 2013 Jan;44(1):59–66.

46

GALEAZZI FRACTURE

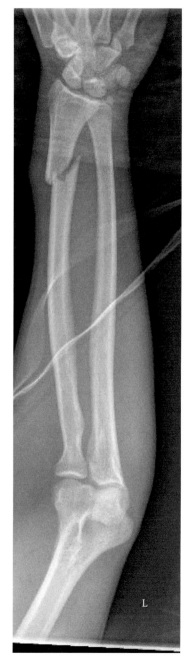
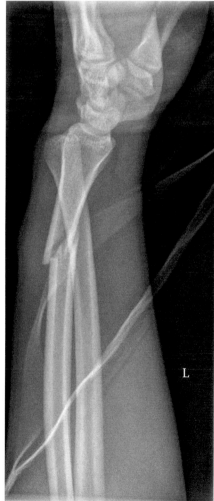

These are the radiographs of a 20-year-old man who fell on his outstretched hand during a rugby match.

1. **Describe the appearances shown in these radiographs.**

   These are an AP and lateral radiographs of the forearm. They show a midshaft diaphyseal fracture of the radius, which is displaced. The distal ulna is also dorsally displaced, indicating an injury to the distal radioulnar joint (DRUJ). This injury pattern is referred to as a *Galeazzi fracture dislocation*.

2. **How would you choose to manage this injury?**

   In a patient who is fit enough to undertake surgery, I would choose to treat this operatively. After obtaining the necessary consent and preoperative work up and under general anaesthesia with prophylactic antibiotics and a proximal arm tourniquet, I would use a modified Henry's approach in order to reduce and fix the radius fracture with a 3.5 mm LC-DC plate. I would operate with image intensifier guidance. Reduction of the radius fracture usually facilitates reduction of the DRUJ but I would check this directly and with the image intensifier. I would also make an assessment of DRUJ stability in the forearm neutral, supinated and pronated positions. If the DRUJ is entirely stable I would allow early active movement. DRUJ instability in either forearm supination or pronation would be treated by splinting the forearm in the forearm position of stability (pronation or supination). If I found gross instability in both supination and pronation then I would percutaneously K-wire the DRUJ in a reduced position in supination. I would use two 2 mm K-wires and I would protect the wires for a period of 6 weeks by placing the patient in a hinged elbow brace to allow flexion and extension but to prevent forearm supination and pronation.

3. **What features on a plain radiograph would make you suspicious of a Galeazzi type injury rather than an isolated diaphyseal fracture of the radius?**

   DRUJ injury is suggested by fracture of the ulnar styloid base, widening of the DRUJ on the PA radiograph, dorsal subluxation of the distal ulna on the lateral radiograph or marked shortening of the radius relative to the ulna. However, the gold standard for assessment is clinical examination of the DRUJ.

4. **What are the stabilisers of the distal radioulnar joint?**

   The distal radioulnar joint is stabilised by bony stabilisers and soft tissue stabilisers. The bony component is provided by the articulation of the distal ulna with the sigmoid notch of the distal radius. The soft tissue stabilisers are a collection of ligamentous structures collectively referred to as the *triangular fibrocartilaginous complex* (TFCC). The individual components are the articular disc or triangular fibrocartilage, meniscal homologue, the ulnolunate and the ulnotriquetral ligaments. The dorsal and volar radioulnar ligaments, the extensor carpi ulnaris sub sheath and the ulnar collateral ligament also stabilise the distal radioulnar joint.

FURTHER READING

Giannoulis FS, Sotereanos DG. Galeazzi fractures and dislocations. *Hand Clin.* 2007 May;23(2):153–163.

Tsismenakis T, Tornetta P III. Galeazzi fractures: Is DRUJ instability predicted by current guidelines? *Injury.* 2016 Jul;47(7):1472–1477.

47

BOTH BONES FOREARM FRACTURE

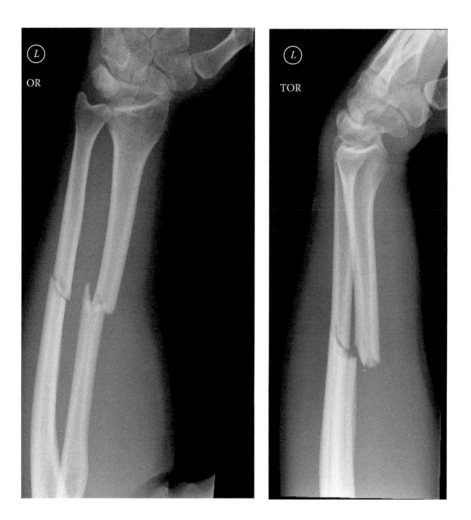

A 32-year-old woman is admitted after a fall from her bicycle. She has an isolated injury to her left upper limb. These are her radiographs.

1. **What do the radiographs show?**

   The radiographs show displaced midshaft diaphyseal fractures of both bones of the left forearm.

2. **How would you treat this injury?**

   I would make a careful patient assessment, completing the history and examination. Particularly, I would look for any open wounds, make an assessment of the soft tissues and the neurovascular status of the limb as well as any suggestion of compartment syndrome. I would ensure that the patient has adequate analgesia and would splint the forearm in an above elbow backslab in 90 degrees of flexion. In an otherwise healthy adult I would plan to treat this injury definitively on the next routine trauma operating list with dynamic compression plating of both fractures using 3.5 mm LC-DC plates.

3. **Ten months after surgery, you are following up this patient in clinic and these are her radiographs. What do they show and what treatment would you advise?**
   These radiographs show that the fracture has been treated operatively with plate fixation. The alignment appears satisfactory; however, there is a persisting delayed or non-union of the ulnar fracture. The radius seems to have united.

   I would complete my assessment of the patient, looking for any persisting symptoms suggestive of delayed union or non-union or infection such as pain, local swelling or erythema. I would take some blood for full blood count and inflammatory markers. I would arrange a CT scan of the forearm to confirm the degree of union of both fractures and if non-union is confirmed in the absence of infection I would advise revision fixation of the non-union with autologous iliac crest bone grafting.

   I would consider the use of a bone stimulator for 6–8 weeks as an interim measure and current guidance suggests that this is appropriate for an established non-union after 9 months. If the screening investigations are suggestive of infection, then I would send peripheral blood and wound samples for culture. I would also perform an initial debridement at which I would sample tissue taken from the non-union site so that targeted antibiotic treatment can be given before definitive grafting is undertaken.

FURTHER READING

NICE medical technology guidance [MTG12]. EXOGEN ultrasound bone healing system for long bone fractures with non-union or delayed healing. 2013. Accessed from https://www.nice.org.uk/guidance/mtg12.

Schulte LM, Meals CG, Neviaser RJ. Management of adult diaphyseal both-bone forearm fractures. *J Am Acad Orthop Surg*. 2014 Jul;22(7):437–446. doi: 10.5435/JAAOS-22-07-437.

48

DISTAL RADIUS FRACTURE

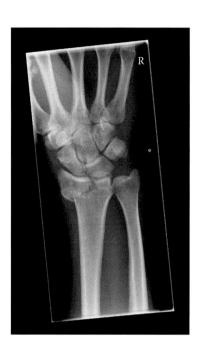
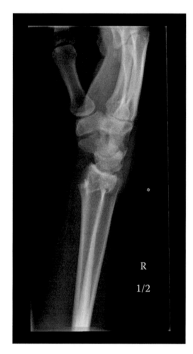

You are called to the emergency department to see a 65-year-old active right hand dominant woman. She tells you that she has fallen, injuring her right wrist. She is neurovascularly intact.

1. **Describe these radiographs.**
   These are an AP and lateral radiograph of the right wrist, which show a dorsally angulated and displaced fracture of the distal radius.

2. **How would you manage this patient?**
   Assuming that this is a closed injury without neurovascular deficit, my treatment would depend on a number of patient-related factors and injury or fracture-related factors. Relevant patient factors include patient biological and physiological age, functional demands of the patient, comorbidities and fitness for surgery. Injury-related factors include any associated neurovascular deficit, open wounds, comminution and potential for instability.

   This is an unstable injury with marked radial shortening as well as dorsal and metaphyseal comminution. I would discuss the benefits of operative versus non-operative treatment with the patient but my advice would be that for an active patient with reasonable functional demands I should perform a careful closed manipulation under Bier's block or sedation would restore length, alignment and also reduce tension on the soft tissues, as well as swelling and tension on local nerves. I would place the patient in a below elbow backslab and check the post manipulation position with x-rays, and if a satisfactory reduction is achieved then I would review the patient at 1 week in the fracture clinic with repeat radiographs.

If the position is maintained, I would complete the cast but I would warn the patient that this injury has a considerable risk of instability and I would review the patient in the fracture clinic after another week in clinic with further radiographs. If the position is maintained, I would treat the patient in a plaster cast for a total of 6 weeks. I would treat the loss of position in the first 2 weeks with surgery and in this situation, I would use a volar locking plate.

3. The fracture redisplaces to the original position within the week. How would you treat this?

I would have a discussion with the patient about the risks and benefits of surgery. In a patient of this age the bone quality is likely to be osteoporotic and fixation with Kirschner wires is less reliable, especially for comminuted fractures. I would choose to treat this fracture with locked volar plating through a modified Henry's approach which would allow early movement and remove the need for plaster cast treatment.

4. What are the radiographic predictors of instability?

Various studies have examined a number of radiographic and patient related predictors of instability. Patient age is consistently agreed as an important patient-related factor. This may be representative of bone quality. Radiographic factors include fracture comminution, radial shortening or ulna variance and an associated fracture of the distal ulna.

FURTHER READING

Costa ML, Achten J, Plant C, Parsons NR, Rangan A, Tubeuf S, Yu G, Lamb SE. UK DRAFFT: A randomised controlled trial of percutaneous fixation with Kirschner wires versus volar locking-plate fixation in the treatment of adult patients with a dorsally displaced fracture of the distal radius. *Health Technol Assess.* 2015 Feb;19(17):1–124.

Henry MH. Distal radius fractures: Current concepts. *J Hand Surg Am.* 2008 Sept;33:1215–1227.

Lafontaine M, Delince P, Hardy D, Simons M. Instability of fractures of the lower end of the radius: Apropos of a series of 167 cases. *Acta Orthop Belg.* 1989 Feb;55:203–216.

Leone J, Bhandari M, Adili A, Mackenzie S, Moro JK, Dunlop RB. Predictors of early and late instability following conservative treatment of extraarticular distal radius fractures. *Arch Orthop Trauma Surg.* 2004 Jan;124:38–41.

Mackenney PJ, McQueen MM, Elton R. Prediction of instability in distal radius fractures. *J Bone Joint Surg Am.* 2006 Sep;88(9):1944–1951.

49

SCAPHOID FRACTURE

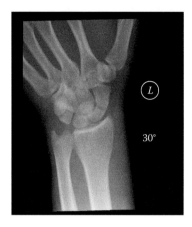
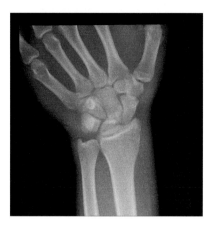

1. **How would you assess for a scaphoid fracture on clinical examination?**
   I would inspect the affected limb for swelling, ecchymosis and any obvious wounds. I would assess for the presence of focal bony and soft tissue tenderness, particularly around the anatomical snuffbox, distal radius and ulna, the scaphoid tubercle and the scapholunate interval. I would perform axial loading of the thumb in order to provoke any symptoms related to base of thumb pathology or scaphoid fracture. I would also assess the active range of wrist movement in particular, looking for pain on the radial and ulnar deviation of the wrist.

2. **Describe these radiographs and the diagnosis.**
   This is a postero-anterior (PA) radiograph of the wrist, as well as a partially supinated oblique view to show the scaphoid en face. The diagnosis is an undisplaced fracture of the scaphoid waist.

   The standard radiographs for a scaphoid fracture include four views of the wrist: The postero-anterior with ulnar deviation, lateral, semi-pronated oblique, and semi-supinated oblique views.

3. **How would you manage this acute, undisplaced scaphoid waist fracture?**
   I would have a discussion with the patient and discuss the pros and cons for operative and non-operative treatment options, thus allowing the patient to make an informed choice.

   For most patients, I would advise conservative management where I would employ a short arm cast with the thumb left free. This allows for the use of the hand and the elbow is not immobilised. Casting for 8 weeks will lead to a union rate of around 90% to 95% of scaphoid waist fractures.

   There is evidence that percutaneous screw fixation offers advantages and in particular that this surgery reduces the time needed for 'return to work' for the patient. I would discuss this with the patient. I would tell the patient that there are additional risks with surgery although these are uncommon. They will be able to use the hand and wrist sooner with operative management and will likely avoid the need to use plaster immobilisation, but they will have to avoid contact sports for a similar period of time. Long-term outcomes and union rates are similar with both treatment options.

4. How would you manage this if it were an acute proximal pole fracture?

There is a very high rate of non-union in proximal pole fractures when managed conservatively and I would generally advise acute fixation of these.

5. What are the other indications for acute fixation of scaphoid fractures?

- Displacement >1 mm
- Scapholunate angle >60 degrees
- Intrascaphoid angle >35 degrees (humpback deformity)
- Fractures associated with perilunate dislocations (high-energy injuries with high chance of non-union)
- Delayed union
- Patient preference (generally reserved for athletes or young manual workers)

FURTHER READING

Scaphoid Waist Internal Fixation for Fractures Trial (SWIFFT). Cast treatment versus surgical fixation of fractures of the scaphoid waist in adults: A multi-centre randomised controlled trial. Accessed from http://www.nets.nihr.ac.uk/projects/hta/113637.

Yin ZG, Zhang JB, Kan SL, Wang P. Treatment of acute scaphoid fractures: Systematic review and meta-analysis. *Clin Orthop.* 2007 July;460:142–151.

50

PERILUNATE DISLOCATION

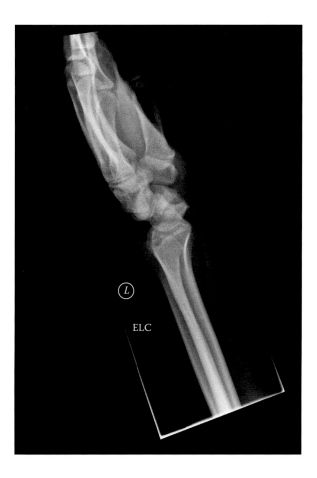

1. Describe this radiograph.

This is a lateral radiograph of the wrist showing a perilunate dislocation. The lateral view shows a dorsal dislocation of the capitate and distal carpal row. The lunate remains in the lunate fossa of the radius owing to its strong ligamentous attachments from the short and the long radiolunate ligaments.

The PA view would show disruption of Gilula's lines and the capitate overlapping the lunate. There are no obvious fractures but I would look closely in order to identify any of the more commonly associated bony injuries, including fractures to the radial styloid, scaphoid, capitate, trapezoid, hamate and ulnar styloid.

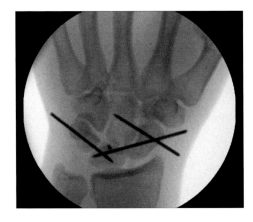

2. How would you manage this injury in the emergency department?

This is a potentially high-energy injury and the patient will require concurrent assessment and treatment as per ATLS guidelines. Specifically for the affected limb, I would perform a circumferential examination to ensure it is a closed injury and assess the neurovascular status of the hand, in particular the median nerve. I would provide the patient with suitable analgesia and arrange for a closed reduction in the emergency department, utilising the Tavernier's manoeuvre (traction, wrist extension with direct thumb pressure on the lunate, followed by wrist flexion) and place the patient in a plaster of Paris below elbow backslab. I would assess for a congruent reduction with AP and lateral radiographs prior to discussing definitive operative management with the patient.

3. How would you classify this injury?

These injuries can be broadly divided into greater arc injuries, which include one or more fractures, or lesser arc injuries, which are purely ligamentous.

As this is a purely ligamentous injury, it would be classified as a lesser arc, with a typical pattern of injury described by Mayfield:

- Stage I – Failure of the scapholunate ligament
- Stage II – Stage I + lunocapitate joint disruption
- Stage III – Stage I + II + lunotriquetral joint disruption (perilunate dislocation)
- Stage IV – Lunate dislocation (usually volar through the space of Poirier – note the high rate of carpal tunnel syndrome)

This patient has sustained a Mayfield stage III lesser arc perilunate dislocation.

4. How would you manage this injury definitively following a satisfactory closed reduction in the emergency department?

I would admit the patient to ward for high elevation with a Bradford sling in addition to providing regular analgesia and regular neurovascular observations. Definitive management would be operative due to the high rate of recurrent dislocation for conservatively managed injuries, but may be considered when other medical reasons contraindicate surgical intervention.

There is no universally accepted operative treatment; however, the principles include fixing associated fractures, repairing the scapholunate ligament and protecting the scapholunate ligament repair.

I would advocate open reduction, K-wire fixation and ligament repair, utilising an open dorsal approach. I would reduce the scapholunate and lunotriquetral joints and maintain reduction with K-wires.

The dorsal incision allows for repair of the dorsal scapholunate ligament (this is stronger than the palmar SL ligament). The ligament repairs are carried out either with suture anchors for ligaments avulsed from bone (most common scenario) or with direct suturing for ligaments torn in their midsubstance. There is no evidence to suggest superior outcomes if the lunotriquetral ligament is also repaired, and this would require a separate volar approach.

K-wires (pictured) should be placed from the triquetrum to the lunate, the scaphoid to the lunate, and the scaphoid to the capitate. These would be buried and removed 8 weeks postoperatively.

Postoperatively, I would place the patient in a cast for 8 weeks at which point the cast and wires could be removed and gentle rehabilitation could begin with a removable splint worn between physiotherapy sessions.

51

LUNATE DISLOCATION

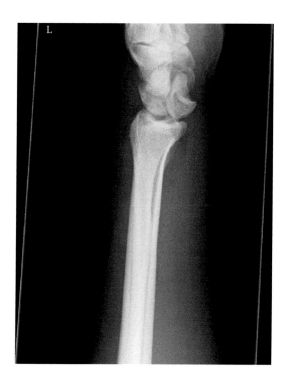

1. **Describe this radiograph. What additional imaging might you request and what would you expect this to show?**

This is a lateral radiograph of the left wrist which shows a volar dislocation of the lunate while the capitate is now articulating with the radius.

I would request a PA view of the wrist and I would scrutinise this to look for malalignment in the carpus and of the radiocarpal axis. I would expect to see interruption of Gilula's lines and the lunate might appear to be 'wedge'- or 'slice of pie'-shaped and overlap the capitate. I would scrutinise the radiographs for any evidence of fractures and or intercarpal widening.

The PA view would likely show disruption of the Gilula's lines, with the capitate appearing to overlap the lunate. One would also look for common bony injuries including the radial styloid, scaphoid, capitate, trapezoid, hamate and ulnar styloid.

2. **How many Gilula lines are there?**

There are three in total:

- The first line is a smooth curve outlining the proximal convex surfaces of the scaphoid, lunate and triquetrum.
- The second line traces the distal concave surfaces of the same bones.
- The third line follows the proximal curvatures of the capitate and hamate.

3. How would you manage this injury in the emergency department?

This is a potentially high-energy injury and I would assess the patient using ATLS guidelines. With respect to this specific limb injury, I would perform a circumferential examination to confirm it is a closed injury and I would assess the neurovascular status of the hand. The median nerve is at greatest risk of injury. I would provide the patient with suitable analgesia and arrange to perform a closed reduction emergently under conscious sedation. I would achieve this by applying longitudinal traction across the wrist with slight wrist extension while applying direct thumb pressure over the lunate from palmar to dorsal. The wrist is then gently flexed and the lunate 'thumbed' back into place. The traction is relaxed and I would place the wrist in a below elbow backslab so that the wrist is immobilised in 10 degrees of palmar flexion. I would confirm the reduction and position in plaster using PA and lateral radiographs.

If closed reduction proves unsuccessful then I would place the patient in a wrist splint and elevate the limb in a Bradford sling to minimise swelling. I would admit the patient and prepare them for open reduction via a palmar carpal tunnel approach and surgical stabilisation to be performed on the next available operating list by an experienced upper limb surgeon.

4. Through what space has the lunate dislocated and what are its boundaries?

The lunate has dislocated through the space of Poirier. This is the space between the long radiolunate and radioscaphoid-capitate ligaments.

5. How would you manage this injury following a satisfactory closed reduction in the emergency department?

I would admit the patient to the ward for high elevation with a Bradford sling, regular analgesia and neurovascular observations. I would advise operative management to restore joint alignment and stability. I would use a dorsal approach to the wrist and carpus. I would realign the proximal carpal row and repair the scapholunate ligament with a suture anchor. I would protect the repair with K-wires across the scapholunate joint and I would also pin the lunotriquetral joint in position with a further K-wire. I would place the patient in a below elbow cast for 8 weeks and I would encourage the patient to maintain finger joint movement during this time. After this period, I would remove the k-wires and start formal rehabilitation with skilled hand therapy.

52

FIGHT BITE

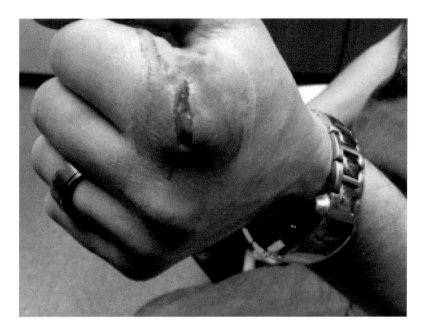

A 28-year-old man presents 72 hours following an injury to his left hand. He seems evasive about the history but finally admits to being involved in a fight.

1. **Can you describe the picture and the underlying injury?**
   This clinical photograph shows a wound over the metacarpophalangeal joint of the index finger of the left hand. Despite the vague history I would be suspicious of a 'fight bite' wound over the MCPJ caused by a penetrating tooth injury. This would potentially extend down to the underlying joint. The injury may cause septic arthritis, in addition to extensor tendon damage, osteochondral injury, associated fractures or osteomyelitis in neglected injuries.

2. **How would you assess the patient in the emergency department?**
   I would take a full history from the patient, with the knowledge that some patients may be reluctant to reveal the full history. I would have a high index of suspicion for a 'fight bite'. I would wish to know hand dominance and occupation, in addition to past medical history and tetanus immunisation status. I would ask the patient if he knew the person he punched and if their bloodborne virus status is known. I would assess for signs of sepsis through observations (looking for pyrexia, tachycardia, tachypnoea and hypotension) in addition to inflammatory markers (white cell count and CRP).

   On examination, I would assess the wound for signs of cellulitis, obvious purulence, tendon rupture and septic arthritis. I would request plain radiographs to assess for underlying fractures and retained tooth fragments.

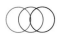

3. How should this injury be managed?

Fight bites invariably warrant operative management due to the potential to develop septic arthritis. I would administer tetanus prophylaxis if indicated and take swabs from the wound prior to starting broad-spectrum intravenous antibiotics in accordance with local microbiology guidelines (co-amoxiclav would be the antibiotic of choice in my unit). The infection is typically polymicrobial but the most common organism cultured from a fight bite is *Staphylococcus aureus*. Gram negative bacteria should also be covered with the antibiotics as *Eikenella corrodens* is often implicated in a fight bite. I would photograph the wound and cover with saline-soaked swabs and a non-adherent dressing.

I would take the patient to theatre for a debridement under general anaesthesia with an arm tourniquet. I would extend the wound to examine the underlying structures, with particular attention being paid to recreating the hand position at the time of injury to examine the underlying tendon and look for penetration of the joint. If the tendon is ruptured, I would tag the ends and not attempt a primary repair at this time. Deep tissue samples should be sent at the time of surgery and I would commence intravenous antibiotic therapy.

I would inspect the joint and irrigate it with copious volumes of normal saline. I would partially close the wound by suturing my wound extensions and applying a sterile, non-adherent dressing. I would instruct the ward to elevate the arm with a Bradford sling and I would reinspect the wound 48 hours postop on the ward and assess the need for further surgery and tendon repair.

53

JERSEY FINGER

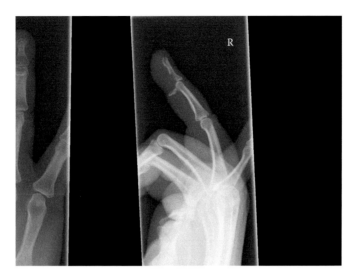

A 22-year-old medical student presents to the emergency department with a painful and swollen ring finger at the distal interphalangeal joint. Forty-eight hours earlier he injured his finger playing for the Edinburgh Medics Rugby Football Club and he thinks the injury occurred whilst tackling an opponent. He managed to finish the game but complains of discomfort and reduced movement in the finger ever since.

1. **What does the picture show?**

   This history would lead me to suspect a 'jersey finger' or 'rugger jersey finger', which is a type of zone 1 flexor tendon injury. These are commonly described in American football players and classically occur when a tackler grabs hold of an opponent's jersey. The distal interphalangeal joint (DIPJ) is forcibly hyperextended while the flexor digitorum profundus (FDP) muscle contracts leading to tendon rupture at its weakest point, the insertion on the distal phalanx.

2. **How would you examine the patient to confirm the diagnosis and what would the radiographs likely show?**

   Inability to flex the DIPJ is suggestive of rupture of the FDP tendon. On inspection, the injured finger may lie in slight extension compared with the other fingers in the resting posture. There may be tenderness on the volar side of the finger and the retracted tendon may be palpable over the proximal phalanx or in the palm.

   I would test FDP function by fixing the middle phalanx in extension preventing flexion at the proximal interphalangeal joint (PIPJ) and asking the patient to attempt to actively flex the finger at the DIPJ. This prevents the action of flexor digitorum superficialis (FDS) and isolates the FDP.

   Radiographs are often normal in a jersey finger injury, although in this case they reveal an avulsion fracture from the base of the distal phalanx.

3. Which finger is most commonly affected and why?

The ring finger. Traditionally, this is thought to be due to its prominence compared with other digits in flexion that may expose it to greater forces during grip. Another theory is that this is down to its restriction to passive extension due to intertendinous connections: The ring finger cannot be fully extended when the middle and small finger MCPJs are flexed to 90 degrees. Ultimately, the predominance of ring finger injuries is likely multifactorial.

4. How are these injuries classified?

Leddy and Packer classified FDP tendon avulsion injuries on the basis of the extent of proximal retraction of the tendon and the type of avulsion. The further the tendon retracts the greater the likelihood of damage to the blood supply owing to rupture of the vincular system, which carries the blood vessels that supply the tendon.

Type I	FDP tendon avulsion with retraction to the palm. Leads to disruption of the vascular supply.
Type II	FDP tendon avulsion with retraction to the distal end of the A2 pulley. The blood supply is only partially disrupted.
Type III	Large bony fragment avulsion, which cannot retract beyond the distal A4 pulley due to its size. The blood supply is intact.

This classification system was modified by Smith with the addition of a type IV injury: This is an unusual combination of a bony avulsion from the distal phalanx and tendon avulsion from the fragment into the palm.

5. How should this injury be managed?

Prompt diagnosis and surgical repair of FDP avulsions is recommended in order to preserve any residual blood supply and also because clinical assessment of the level of injury is inexact.

Non-operative management is rare and is reserved for cases where surgery is contraindicated because of patient co-morbidities.

Type I injury: The tendon has retracted into the palm, and it is presumed to be avascular and vulnerable to contraction. Early intervention (by 7–10 days) with primary repair will achieve the best outcomes.

Two incisions are required to repair type I injuries. The first, a Bruner-type incision, is made over the FDP tendon insertion site. The second incision is made over the A1 pulley or proximal to this to retrieve the tendon. Once the retracted tendon is identified it can be passed back through the finger pulley system using a paediatric feeding tube. A distal pull-through suture tied over a button technique is widely used, but these can deform the nail plate and are vulnerable to infection. Failure can be due to the reliance on early healing of the tendon to the bone. Outcomes of the use of bone anchors have been reported with favourable outcomes.

In type II injuries, the tendon is maintained within the sheath by an intact long vinculum. With presumed partial preservation of the blood supply, contraction of the tendon is less likely. Repair is recommended within 3 weeks and the techniques used are similar for type I injuries.

Type III injuries have a large bone fragment which prevents proximal retraction beyond the distal end of the A4 pulley. Due to the minimal tendon retraction, primary surgical repair can be performed up to 6 weeks after the injury.

Treatment depends on the fragment size. Fracture repair can be performed using K-wires or miniature screw fixation, although transosseous sutures can also be used. Very small or extra-articular bone fragments can be excised without shortening the tendon, allowing the use of tendon-to-bone repair techniques (discussed previously).

Type IV injuries require a combination of techniques used for types I–III injuries. Again, treatment depends on the size and the intra-articular nature of the bone fragment. As in type I injuries, prompt tendon repair is required (by 7–10 days).

Hand therapy is essential for a good outcome, with early active mobilisation preferred as long as the surgical repair is robust enough to tolerate this.

It is not uncommon for patients to present late or for diagnosis to be delayed. In such cases, reconstruction options include two-stage tendon grafting or fusion of the DIPJ.

SECTION III
GENERAL TRAUMA PRINCIPLES

54

ATLS

All polytrauma patients and trauma patients with high-energy injuries should be assessed according to advanced trauma life support (ATLS) principles. You may be asked to describe a detailed ATLS assessment of a patient prior to moving onto a specific orthopaedic or extremity injury. It is absolutely essential that you are confident with this routine system for assessment.

You are called to the emergency department as part of the trauma team to see a patient who was involved in a high-speed RTA. He was the restrained driver in a head-on collision with a tree. He was immobilised at the scene and taken straight to the emergency department. He is talking, but confused, tachycardic and hypotensive.

1. **How would you manage this injury?**

I would manage this injury in the emergency department according to ATLS principles with concurrent assessment and resuscitation undertaken by the whole trauma team. I would start by assessing the airway with cervical spine control. The cervical spine must be immobilised with all three of a hard collar, sandbags and tape. If the patient is talking, he has a patent airway; if not, it must be formally assessed with the look/listen/feel approach. This is done by looking in the mouth for foreign bodies or trauma, attempting suction if appropriate, listening for abnormal breath sounds such as stridor or hoarseness of the voice and feeling for breath on your cheek as you look for chest wall movements.

Moving onto breathing and ventilation, I would administer high-flow oxygen using a non-rebreathe mask as other members of the team are attaching monitoring at this stage to determine pulse from a three-lead ECG, blood pressure, oxygen saturations, respiratory rate and temperature. An inspection/palpation/percussion/auscultation approach is taken, looking for any obvious chest injuries such as open wounds or flail segments. One would also look for respiratory distress and symmetrical chest wall movement. I would look for symmetrical chest wall movement and any evidence of respiratory distress. I would palpate to assess for the central position of the trachea and any subcutaneous emphysema. I would percussion and auscultate to confirm good bilateral air entry and to identify an obvious pneumothorax or haemothorax.

Moving on to circulation with haemorrhage control, I would gain IV access with two large-bore cannulae into the antecubital fossas, taking blood for FBC, U&Es, LFTs, glucose, lactate, coagulation and cross-match for at least four units of bloods. I would then commence appropriate resuscitation as per my hospital's major haemorrhage protocol* before moving on to look for any obvious source of bleeding in the chest, abdomen, pelvis, long bones or floor. I would apply a pelvic binder (although

---

* Traditional ATLS teaching at this stage is to administer 2L of warmed Ringer's lactate (Hartmann's). Modern teaching has moved on from this, with targeted resuscitation and a move towards the replacement of 'like with like', replacing lost blood with O-negative blood products prior to group specific and, later, fully cross-matched blood. For the exam, it would be advisable to have an example from your own hospital/local trauma unit, with most units moving towards a 1:1:1 protocol (1 unit red cell concentrate (RCC), 1 unit of fresh frozen plasma (FFP) and 1 unit of pooled platelets). The local fixed ratio protocol should be changed to a protocol guided by laboratory results as soon as possible (see below for an example).

ideally this would have been done pre-hospital for any polytrauma patient with evidence of hypovolaemic shock) and I would request a trauma series of c-spine, chest and pelvic radiographs at this stage, as long as they don't get in the way of resuscitation.

Moving onto disability, I would assess the pupils, perform an AVPU and GCS score and D (don't ever forget blood glucose).

Environment/exposure is next, where the patient is completely undressed, taking care to prevent hypothermia and respect privacy, and they are then log-rolled to allow for inspection of the patient's back and to remove the spinal board. Consideration can be given at this stage to urinary catheterisation/need for further imaging/surgery and ultimate location of the patient, that is, ward/HDU/ITU, prior to moving onto the secondary survey. Imaging in the form of a CT scan (from the vertex of the skull to the symphysis pubic) with intravenous contrast is obtained if the patient is stable enough to be transferred to CT.

Should the patient deteriorate at any stage I would return to reassess the airway with cervical spine control and assess the patient again in a logical order.

In my hospital, patients with active or severe bleeding have their resuscitation managed in line with a major haemorrhage protocol, which is summarised here.

The major haemorrhage protocol should be activated in the context of ongoing severe bleeding or haemorrhagic shock:

- Activate major haemorrhage protocol.
- Use O-negative blood as necessary (this is usually present in A&E and the-atre recovery). Group-specific blood (ABO + RhD grouping) generally takes 15–20 minutes; fully cross-matched blood 30–40 minutes.
- Where no results are available, order six units of RCC and four units of FFP. If bleeding persists and still no blood results, order a further four units of RCC and four units of FFP, in addition to one unit of platelets and two pools of cryoprecipitate.
- Rotational thromboelastometry (ROTEM) should be used where available to guide resuscitation.
- Tranexamic acid has been shown to reduce the risk of death in bleeding trauma patients (CRASH 2 trial). It is given as a 1 g bolus over 10 minutes followed by a 1 g infusion over 8 hours.
- Once results are available, target driven resuscitation should be performed as follows.

Parameter	Aim for	Intervention
Hb	>8 g/dL	
PT & APTT	Normal	Transfuse 4 units FFP if APTT or PT ratio >1.5
Fibrinogen	>1 g/L	Transfuse 2 units of pooled cryoprecipitate if <1
Platelets	>75 × 10⁹/L	Transfuse 1 unit of platelets if <75 (2 units if <30)

2. What are signpost injuries?

There are injuries which should alert the clinician to the possibility of other associated injuries. Examples include:

- Spinal fractures: Where a spinal fracture is present, there is a 10% possibility of a spinal fracture at another level.

- Scapular fractures: These rare injuries represent a high-energy injury and one should be mindful of potential injury to the thorax, for example lung contusion/haemothorax/pneumothorax.
- Sternal fractures: Similar to scapular fractures, these are rare and are indicative of a high-energy injury. Care must be taken to rule out associated thoracic injuries.
- Calcaneal fractures: These are generally sustained from an axial load injury. This should alert the clinician to the possibility of other axial load injuries, for example, pilon, tibial plateau, femur, hip, acetabulum/pelvis and spine. The most frequent associated injury with one calcaneal fracture however is a contralateral calcaneal fracture.
- Knee dislocation: These are frequently associated with a common peroneal nerve injury. There is also a risk of damage to the popliteal artery.
- Hip dislocation (posterior): This may be associated with a sciatic nerve injury or a posterior wall acetabular fracture. If sustained following a 'dashboard' injury, there is a risk of knee ligamentous injury, patella fracture or a femoral fracture.
- Femoral shaft: In the young, there is an 8–10% rate of concurrent femoral neck fractures.

FURTHER READING

National Institute for Health and Clinical Excellence (NICE). Major trauma: Assessment and initial management. 2016. Accessed 1 May 2016 from https://www.nice.org.uk/guidance/ng39.

55

OPEN FRACTURE

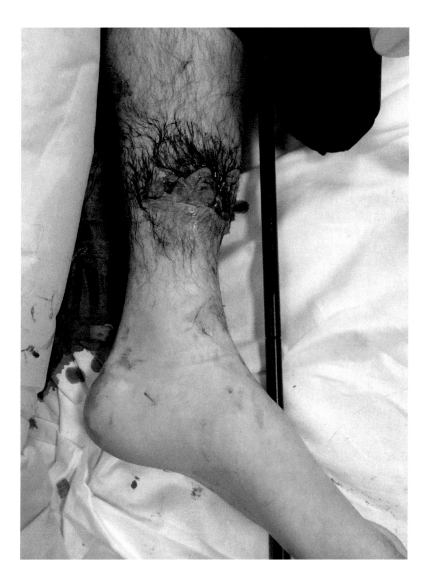

1. **Describe what you see and your initial management in the emergency department.**
   This is a clinical photograph revealing an open tibial fracture. There is a large transverse wound over the medial border of the tibia with exposed bone protruding. There is obvious periosteal stripping and contusion to the surrounding skin.

   This patient requires management in accordance with ATLS principles as it is likely a high-energy injury with potential for other more life-threatening injuries to be present.

Specifically for the open fracture, I would perform a full neurovascular examination of the affected limb. I would remove any obvious contamination from the wound, photograph it, and then cover it with a saline-soaked swab. I would provide analgesia, and splint the limb as well as obtain radiographs if not already performed.

I would give antibiotics as per local microbiology protocols (the BOAST guidelines suggest cefuroxime 1.5 g IV) and assess the need for tetanus prophylaxis.

2. **When should the patient go to theatre and what will you plan to do?**

The current consensus favours prudent early surgery within the first 24 hours. The old '6-hour rule' was based on animal experiments from the 1890s, and the well-known Lower Extremity Assessment Project (LEAP) study* found no difference in infection rates when open fractures were managed within 6 hours or 24 hours. The BOAST guidelines recommend urgent surgery if there is a vascular injury or the wound is heavily contaminated by marine, agricultural or sewage matter.

Assuming there is no vascular injury, this injury is best managed during daytime hours with combined orthopaedic and plastic surgery input. The wound will be thoroughly debrided in a systematic fashion from outside to in, including skin, fat, fascia, muscle and bone. Non-viable skin should be excised, but any skin that is of dubious viability may be left for later assessment/debridement, unlike necrotic muscle which is implicated in infection and must be removed. Muscle can be assessed utilising the 4 Cs (colour, consistency, contractility, cut [does it bleed?]).

I would deliver the bone ends and debride these, in addition to removing any devitalised bone which fails the 'tug test'. I would wash out the wound and fracture with 6 litres of warmed normal saline. I would then stabilise the fracture provisionally using an external fixator or definitively with an intramedullary nail if I agree with my plastic surgery colleague that definitive surgery is safe and wound closure or coverage can be achieved. Antibiotics would be given at the time of surgery and continued for 72 hours or until wound closure, whichever occurs soonest.

3. **What is your biggest concern in the postoperative period and how would you monitor for this?**

With any high-energy fracture, particularly of the tibia, I would have a high index of suspicion for compartment syndrome. Although the open fracture has created a rent in the fascia, this in no way precludes the development of compartment syndrome. Diagnosis of compartment syndrome is a clinical one, but this requires a high index of suspicion in all staff members looking after the patient. Patients who are unconscious or obtunded warrant continuous pressure monitoring with a slit catheter as used for arterial pressure monitoring. Continuous pressure monitoring of the anterior compartment is a useful adjunct to clinical diagnosis, whereby the ΔP is calculated by subtracting the intracompartmental pressure from the diastolic blood pressure. A persistently low ΔP, that is, <30 mmHg, is diagnostic of early compartment syndrome. A caveat to continuous pressure monitoring of the anterior compartment is that one must remain vigilant to the possibility of compartment

---

* LEAP study: This was a multicentre prospective observational study which has published numerous papers since its conception. It identified 601 patients with severe, limb-threatening lower extremity injuries from eight level I trauma centres in the United States and followed them up prospectively for a number of outcomes. Several publications have come from the data collected and the main findings include:
- No difference in infection rate for open fractures managed within 6 hours or within 6 to 24 hours.
- No scoring system was predictive of the need for amputation.
- Loss of plantar sensation is not an absolute indication for amputation.

syndrome developing within the deep posterior compartment, which may give falsely reassuring readings in the anterior compartment.

4. How would you treat compartment syndrome?
I would perform an emergency two-incision, four-compartment fasciotomy of the lower leg. (See Chapter 73.)

5. How soon should you aim for soft tissue coverage and what options are available?
The BOAST guidelines suggest that soft tissue coverage is ideally performed within 72 hours. Options include primary closure, which is an acceptable option when there has been a thorough debridement and soft tissue coverage is possible without tension.

Other options are described by way of the plastic surgery reconstructive ladder. This includes primary closure and healing by secondary intention, escalating to a free flap.

If an open wound involves loss of skin and subcutaneous tissue, but has a base of healthy muscle, fascia, or tendon sheath, granulation tissue will form on the base and a split-thickness skin graft (STSG) can be applied, or the wound can be allowed to heal by secondary intention.

Bare bone, exposed blood vessels, nerves and tendons (without paratenon) all are harmed by desiccation and do not support granulation tissues and STSG. These tissues should not be left exposed, and should be kept moist with appropriate dressings prior to definitive cover.

Reconstructive options	Examples
Healing by secondary intention	–
Primary closure	–
Delayed primary closure	–
STSG	–
FTSG (full thickness skin graft)	Small grafts: Medial forearm and volar wrist crease Large grafts: Lower abdomen and groin
Local flaps	Axial flaps, rotational flaps, rhomboid flaps, V-Y advancement flaps
Rotational muscle flaps	Gastrocnemius rotational flap, soleus rotational flap
Free flaps	Fasciocutaenous/musculocutaneous/osteocutaneous

Regarding flaps for soft tissue coverage of a tibial fracture specifically, the following acts as a guide to treatment options:

- Proximal third tibial defect – Gastrocnemius rotational flap
- Middle third tibial defect – Soleus rotational flap
- Distal third tibial defect – Free flap
- Large defect – Latissimus dorsi
- Smaller defect – Radial forearm
  - Sural artery fasciocutaneous flap

6. How can you grade open fractures?
Open fractures are most commonly graded using the Gustillo and Anderson classification. The original classification from 1976 was based on their experience of

1025 long bone open fractures. Their initial paper proposed a classification system split into grade I, grade II and grade III, but grade III open fractures were highly variable in their pattern of injury and outcomes such as infection. In 1984, Gustillo, Mendoza and Williams modified their initial classification system to include three subtypes in the grade III open fracture and is what orthopaedic surgeons today refer to as the Gustillo and Anderson classification.

Grade I	An open fracture with a clean wound <1cm
Grade II	An open fracture with a wound >1cm but without extensive soft tissue damage or periosteal stripping
Grade III	The following situations warrant automatic grade III classification: • High-energy injury • Gunshot wound • Heavy contamination • Farmyard contamination • Open segmental fracture • Delay to treatment >8 hours • Arterial injury requiring repair IIIa – An open fracture with extensive soft tissue damage but adequate soft tissue coverage IIIb* – An open fracture with extensive soft tissue loss and periosteal stripping IIIc – An open fracture with an associated arterial injury requiring repair

* There is confusion amongst trainees when it comes to the IIIb subtype of open fractures.

In 1994, Brumback and Jones, after conducting a survey of 245 orthopaedic surgeons, concluded that 'interobserver agreement with use of the Gustilo–Anderson classification system for open fractures is moderate to poor'.

In response to that paper, Gustilo wrote in a letter to the editor of the *Journal of Bone and Joint Surgery* (American volume):

Soft-tissue injury is probably the number-one factor in the classification of open fractures. With type I, II, and IIIA fractures, there is enough soft-tissue coverage for delayed primary skin closure or skin-grafting overlying the bone to be recommended. With type IIIB open fractures, after debridement and irrigation of the fracture, the use of local or free vascular flaps is essential because of extensive soft-tissue injury, exposed bone, and periosteal stripping.

More interestingly, as a reply to that letter, Brumback and Jones wrote in the same journal:

With regard to soft-tissue closure, although type IIIB injuries often need full-thickness soft-tissue coverage, it is only in this individual classification that the type of soft-tissue closure helps the examiner to determine the type of open fracture. Even though Dr. Gustilo states that local or freely vascularized flaps are essential in the treatment of type IIIB fractures, this criterion was not part of the definition of the IIIB subtype published in 1984. This exemplifies another criticism of the classification of Gustilo and Anderson: it has been so widely published, frequently with modifications, that even the specific definitions of each type are no longer universal.

To summarise, when describing the original classification, one frequently quotes the 1984 open fracture classification which is in fact a modification of the 1976 paper. Type IIIb is described in the previous table and the need for a flap is not part of the classification system.

FURTHER READING

Brumback RJ, Jones AL. Interobserver agreement in the classification of open fractures of the tibia. The results of a survey of two hundred and forty-five orthopaedic surgeons. *J Bone Joint Surg Am.* 1994 Aug;76(8):1162–1166.

Gustilo RB. Letter to the editor. *J Bone Joint Surg Am.* 1995 Aug;77(8):1291–1292.

56

DAMAGE CONTROL ORTHOPAEDICS

A 28-year-old man is brought to the emergency department after a road traffic accident in which the car he was driving collided with a truck at high speed.

Following his initial treatment in the emergency department he has been intubated because of his reduced level of consciousness and his initial assessment has identified pulmonary contusions, a left sided pneumothorax, some frontal cerebral contusions, bilateral femoral fractures and an open left tibial fracture.

1. **How would you proceed with his resuscitation?**

   This patient is severely injured and will require the attention of a skilled trauma team. He should be treated along ATLS principles with attention to life-threatening injuries and while the system is sequential, the use of a team allows concurrent activity. Active haemorrhage should be controlled and blood products replaced. He should have intravenous access established and a chest drain sited for the pneumothorax. The limbs should be assessed for evidence of haemorrhage, extremity injury and vascular status. The open wound at the tibia should be inspected, gross contamination should be removed, a photograph taken and saline soaked gauze applied. Intravenous antibiotics, usually a cephalosporin, should be administered as well as tetanus toxoid. Spinal precautions should be maintained until the spine can be reliably clinically and radiographically cleared in order to prevent future disability. A trauma CT should be performed examining the head, cervical spine, chest, abdomen and pelvis. If there is any question over the vascular supply to the limbs then a CT angiogram can be performed additionally to identify any vascular injury to the lower limb. The limbs can be splinted temporarily in box splints or plaster to allow transfer.

   The initial resuscitation aims to address life-threatening injuries, stabilise the patient and to normalise abnormal physiology, in particular the lethal triad of hypothermia, coagulopathy and acidosis so that definitive treatment can be undertaken. A decision would be made by the trauma team leader and the neurosurgeons as to whether clinical assessment would suffice or whether an intracranial pressure monitoring device should be placed. Additional monitoring and treatment lines can be placed as required and ventilatory support provided. Resuscitation can be continued in the operating theatre or intensive care unit as appropriate.

2. **Can you tell me about the concepts that would guide your treatment for this patient?**

   The care of the polytraumatised patient has been based on the concepts of early total care where the patient receives early definitive care for all injuries or damage control surgery where temporising initial life and limb saving treatments are undertaken, using external fixators, plaster of Paris, splints and traction for fracture care followed by later definitive treatments. These concepts relate to the pathophysiology of major trauma where the patient undergoes an initial systemic response at the time of injury followed by a further systemic inflammatory response between days 2 and 4 following the initial injury. This is a period where they are at particular risk of pulmonary and systemic complications. Prolonged surgery or major surgery in this period may exacerbate this inflammatory response with poor outcomes and so, for selected patients, there is evidence that a temporising damage control approach is the best treatment strategy.

Early total care is appropriate for patients who are stable as well as unstable patients who respond to initial resuscitation. Patients who are in extremis should be treated with damage control principles. Patients in an intermediate clinical group are referred to as 'borderline'. Serum lactate and the trend in this measurement have been shown to be a good marker of suitability for early total care for these borderline patients. A serum lactate of less than 2 mmol/litre is ideal and a serum level greater than 2.5 mmol/litre has been associated with a poorer response to resuscitation, reduced perfusion and worse outcomes with early total care.

There has been some more recent evidence to suggest that most polytrauma patients actually benefit from early definitive fracture fixation and a new concept of early appropriate care is developing from the two original ideas of damage control and early total care. Early appropriate care is based on the philosophy that early care has been shown to be beneficial for most patients and that patient selection should be based on an individual patient assessment of the presenting patient state and their response to resuscitation.

3. How would you prioritise his orthopaedic injuries for treatment?
Once the patient is optimised for surgery I would ideally plan to treat all limb injuries in one sitting but this would be dependent on the condition of the patient and any change in his condition perioperatively.

I would position the patient on a radiolucent fracture table and proceed to debride and stabilise the tibia fracture first. Depending on the condition of the wound, soft tissues, fracture after debridement and the patient overall, I would consider siting an intrameduallary nail but if there was any concern I would apply an external fixtator to the tibia.

If the patient condition permitted continued surgery then I would proceed to perform bilateral retrograde femoral nail fixation. This has the advantage for the polytraumatised patient that repeated patient re-positioning is not required. If the patient condition does not permit intramedullary nailing then I would apply mono-lateral external fixators to both femoral fractures deferring definitive fixation until the patient was stable enough to tolerate this.

FURTHER READING

Giannoudis PV. Surgical priorities in damage control in polytrauma. *J Bone Joint Surg Br.* 2003 May;85(4):478–483. Review.

Giannoudis PV, Giannoudi M, Stavlas P. Damage control orthopaedics: Lessons learned. *Injury.* 2009 Nov;40 Suppl 4:S47–52.

Nahm NJ, Como JJ, Wilber JH, Vallier HA. Early appropriate care: Definitive stabilization of femoral fractures within 24 hours of injury is safe in most patients with multiple injuries. *J Trauma.* 2011 Jul;71(1):175–185.

Pape HC, Grimme K, Van Griensven M, Sott AH, Giannoudis P, Morley J, Roise O, Ellingsen E, Hildebrand F, Wiese B, Krettek C, EPOFF Study Group. Impact of intramedullary instrumentation versus damage control for femoral fractures on immunoinflammatory parameters: Prospective randomized analysis by the EPOFF Study Group. *J Trauma.* 2003 Jul;55(1):7–13.

57

GUNSHOT INJURY

A 16-year-old male is brought to the emergency department after a reported gunshot injury. He has a wound to the forearm that has been dressed and splinted by the ambulance service.

1. Describe your management of this patient in the emergency department.

This patient would be received in the emergency department by the trauma team and would be treated along ATLS guidelines. The patient should be fully exposed to ensure that any other occult injuries are detected and entry or exit wounds can be clearly identified. The obvious wound should be inspected for signs of obvious major or catastrophic haemorrhage which should be controlled with direct pressure, dressings or a tourniquet if necessary. Any field tourniquets should be exchanged for pneumatic tourniquets. Wounds should be photographed before they are redressed with simple saline-soaked gauze dressings and any obvious contamination removed at the time.

A careful assessment of the neurovascular status is made, the patient is given analgesia as well as prophylactic antibiotics and tetanus immunoglobulin and then the limb is splinted in an above elbow backslab. I would then arrange plain radiographs to include the elbow and wrist. I would complete the assessment with a careful secondary survey. General Medical Council guidance is that all gunshot injuries should be notified to the police.

2. These are the radiographs for this patient. How would you propose to treat this injury?

These are AP and lateral radiographs of the left forearm which show a segmental fracture of the ulna and some foreign material likely to be shrapnel. The clinical photograph shows a wound over the forearm. The degree of soft tissue injury will relate to the energy or velocity of the gunshot and there is the potential for significant injury, cavitation and the introduction of foreign matter into the wound with a high-energy injury.

I would advise operative treatment and would undertake a wound debridement, extending the skin wound longitudinally and excising any necrotic or questionable tissue. I would undertake this with a senior plastic surgeon in attendance. I would send multiple samples for microbiology study, remove any foreign material and shrapnel and irrigate the wound thoroughly with 9 litres of warmed saline, ensuring that I had explored the extent of the injury track. The debridement would include all tissue layers down to and including bone. Following debridement, I would determine whether to apply a plaster cast, external fixator or temporising intramedullary wire in order to confer temporary bony stability. With the plastic surgeon, I would consider whether the wound could and should be primarily closed following debridement or whether graft or flap coverage or even delayed staged treatment would be more appropriate.

I would continue intravenous antibiotics for 72 hours or until initial microbiology results are available for contaminated wounds but would otherwise stop antibiotics following wound closure or coverage. For contaminated wounds or those where it is judged that staged treatment is most appropriate, I would return to the operating theatre for a second look and further debridement with the potential for wound closure or coverage after 48 hours.

FURTHER READING

Burg A, Nachum G, Salai M, Haviv B, Heller S, Velkes S, Dudkiewicz I. Treating civilian gunshot wounds to the extremities in a level 1 trauma center: Our experience and recommendations. *Isr Med Assoc J.* 2009 Sep;11(9):546–551.

Sathiyakumar V, Thakore RV, Stinner DJ, Obremskey WT, Ficke JR, Sethi MK. Gunshot-induced fractures of the extremities: A review of antibiotic and debridement practices. *Curr Rev Musculoskelet Med.* 2015 Sep;8(3):276–289.

58

SCREWS

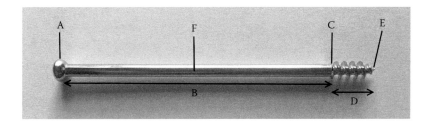

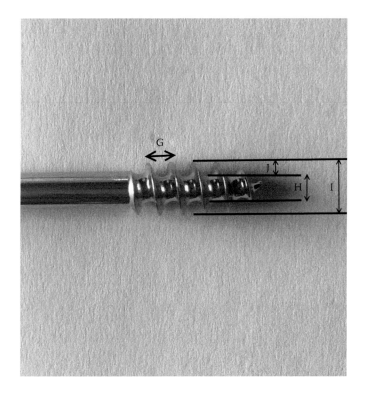

1. What is a screw and what is the function of a screw?

A screw is a mechanical device which converts a rotational force (torque) into a linear movement. Its function is to connect two or more objects by compressing them together.

2. What are the names of the different parts labelled above?

- A – Head
- B – Shank
- C – Run out (this is the area where screws tend to break)

- D – Thread
- E – Tip
- F – Shaft
- G – Pitch
- H – Core diameter/minor diameter
- I – Thread diameter/major diameter
- J – Thread depth

3. Can you tell me the function of the following parts of a screw?

- Head – This provides an area for attachment of a screwdriver and is designed to prevent slip and to improve directional control. It also acts to prevent forward motion of the screw when it is fully seated against bone. Hexagonal head recess design is the most common.
- Flutes – These are present in self-tapping screws and they provide a route for the removal of swarf (bone debris).
- Pitch – This is the distance between threads. It is the same as the distance advanced for every single (360 degrees) turn of the screw.
- Core – The size of the core determines the strength of screw and its fatigue resistance. The size of the drill bit used is equal to the core diameter.
- Threads – Thread depth is half of the difference between thread diameter and core diameter. The thread depth determines the amount of contact with the bones, which in turn determines the resistance to pull out.

4. What is the difference between tensile strength and pullout strength in relation to screws?

The tensile strength of a screw is its resistance to breaking. This is proportional to the core diameter squared.

The pullout strength of a screw depends on the outer diameter of the threads and the area of the threads in contact with the bone. This is the effective thread depth (J in the picture above) and this is proportional to the pullout strength.

5. What type of screw is pictured here?

This is a partially threaded, cancellous screw.

6. How does the pictured screw differ from a locking bolt used with an intramedullary nail?

A locking bolt has superior rotational stability to a screw owing to its wide core diameter. It is particularly useful in osteoporotic bone of the distal femur to prevent the 'broomstick in a trashcan' phenomenon.

7. What drill sizes are required to insert a small fragment cortical screw and a large fragment cortical screw in order for them to act as lag screws?

A lag screw requires two different drill sizes in order to create a gliding hole (near cortex) and a threaded hole (far cortex) as per AO techniques.

A small fragment screw has a major diameter/thread diameter of 3.5 mm and a minor diameter/core diameter of 2.5 mm. This therefore requires:
- 3.5 mm drill bit (silver) for the gliding hole
- 2.5 mm drill bit (gold) for the threaded hole

A large fragment screw has a major diameter/thread diameter of 4.5 mm and a minor diameter/core diameter of 3.2 mm. This therefore requires:

- 4.5 mm drill bit for the gliding hole
- 3.2 mm drill bit for the threaded hole

AO teaching suggests using a standard screw (i.e. not self-tapping) when inserting a lag screw as self-tapping screws can readily angle incorrectly and they will cut a new path and destroy already cut thread. The taps that are used are the same size as the drill bit for the gliding hole.

8. What is the difference between a cortical screw and a cancellous screw?

Cortical screws:

- Smaller pitch
- Greater number of threads
- Thread diameter to core diameter ratio is less
- Designed to have better purchase in cortical bone
- Fully threaded
- Blunt tip

Cancellous screws:

- Greater thread depth
- Larger pitch
- Thread diameter to core diameter ratio is greater
- Designed to have better purchase in the cancellous bone
- Fully or partially threaded
- Corkscrew tip

9. What is the working length of a screw?

This is the length of bone traversed by a screw. In very osteoporotic bones, which typically present a thin cortex or a bone segment under high torsional loading, the use of bicortical screws is mandatory to enhance the working length of the screws, which in turn increases their torsional stiffness. (NB: Despite similar terminology which can lead to confusion, this is an entirely different concept from working length of a nail.)

59

PLATES

1. How is plate strength determined?

Plate strength is defined by the formula BH^3. B is the width; H is height (or thickness). Therefore, the rigidity (bending stiffness) of the plate is proportional to the thickness of the plate to the power of 3.

2. What different functions can a plate provide?

- Bridging: In a comminuted fracture, the plate can bridge the fragment to allow restoration of length, rotation and alignment.
- Buttress: Generally used in the periarticular region. When placed at the apex of the fracture, they prevent displacement of the fracture by shear forces.
- Compression: This can be achieved in several manners:
    1. A lag screw through the plate.
    2. An eccentrically placed screw through the hole of a dynamic compression plate (DCP). There is a potential of 1.8 mm of glide when two holes are compressed, producing up to 600N of compression.
    3. An external compression device, for example, a Verbrugge clamp or AO articulated compression device.
    4. Overbending the plate so there is a small gap between the plate and the bone at the level of the fracture will achieve compression of both the near and far cortex and produce absolute stability.
- Neutralisation: This protects a lag screw from torsional, shear and bending forces.
- Tension band: A plate may be placed on the tension side of the bone to act as a tension band. When the bone is loaded, the plate converts tension into compression at the far cortex.

3. What type of bone healing will occur when a lag screw and neutralisation plate has been used?

Where there has been anatomical reduction and interfragmentary compression, this can achieve absolute stability (no motion between fracture surfaces under functional load). This will lead to direct bone healing (also known as primary bone healing) if the gap between bony fragments is less than 0.01 mm and interfragmentary strain is less than 2%.

Under these conditions, cutting cones are formed at the ends of the osteons closest to the fracture site. The tips of the cutting cones consist of osteoclasts, which cross the fracture line, generating longitudinal cavities at a rate of 50–100 µm/day.

These cavities are filled with blood vessels and osteoblasts, which lay down lamellar bone in the form of new osteons. This process may take many months and is difficult to see on a radiograph due to the lack of callus formation.

4. What type of bone healing will occur when a plate is used as a bridging plate?

When a plate is used as a bridging plate, bone healing will take the form of indirect (secondary) bone healing. This same form of bone healing occurs with cast treatment, IM nails and external fixation. There are four stages.

Stage 1 – Haematoma and Inflammation – Week 1

Haematoma from the ruptured blood vessels forms a fibrin clot. The clotting cascade and complement system are both activated. Macrophages, neutrophils and platelets release several cytokines, including PDGF, TNF-Alpha, TGF-Beta, IL-1, 6, 10, and 12.

There is angiogenesis and recruitment of fibroblasts, mesenchymal cells and osteoprogenitor cells as the haematoma is replaced by granulation tissue, which can tolerate the greatest strain before failure. Necrotic bone ends are resorbed by osteoclasts and other devitalised tissue is removed by macrophages.

Stage 2 – Soft Callus – Weeks 2–4

The granulation tissue formed during stage 1 is replaced by fibrous tissue due to the action of fibroblasts and chondroblasts which lay down cartilage (type II collagen). The mechanical environment drives differentiation of either osteoblastic (stable environment) or chondryocytic (unstable environment) lineages of cells. Cartilage production provides provisional stabilisation.

Stage 3 – Hard Callus – 1–4 months

Soft callus is resorbed by chondroclasts and osteoblasts produce osteoid, which is then mineralised to form woven bone (hard callus). The conversion of soft callus to hard callus is called endochondral ossification.

Stage 4 – Remodelling – Up to several years

Once the fracture has united, the hard callus (woven bone) is replaced with hard, dense lamellar bone by a process of osteoclastic resorption followed by osteoblastic bone formation. This is the same process seen during routine skeletal turnover. The bone assumes a configuration and shape based on stresses acting upon it (Wolff's law).

Electric fields may play a role in Wolff's law. The compression side is electronegative and stimulates osteoblast formation; the tension side is electropositive and simulates osteoclasts.

60

NAILS AND EXTERNAL FIXATORS

1. **How do IM nails and external fixators differ with regard to load bearing and their moment arm?**

   This depends on the fracture type. For AO type A and B fractures with cortical contact, the IM nail or external fixator is load sharing as there is some cortical contact between the main fracture fragments. In a type C fracture, the nail or external fixator is load bearing.

   Although a plate has a short moment arm when fixed to bone, an IM nail is placed down the centre of the intramedullary canal, such that the anatomical axis of the bone is collinear to the long axis of the IM nail. This results in a negligible moment arm and therefore increased stability. An external fixator has the longest moment arm of all three devices given its distance away from the bone.

2. **What different designs of IM nail do you know and what effect do these differences have on performance and stiffness?**

   IM nails come in many different designs. They can be cannulated or solid, slotted or non-slotted, cylindrical or clover leaf-shaped. Cannulated nails are less stiff than solid nails, but can be inserted over a guide wire and allow for deformation during insertion, which makes them less likely to lead to a blow out. Also, micro-motion at the fracture site will encourage secondary/indirect bone healing, which is how fractures heal when treated with IM nails.

   Slotted nails decrease the torsional stiffness as well as bending stiffness and are rarely used these days. Clover leaf-shaped nails are of increased stiffness compared to cylindrical nails.

3. **What is the working length of an intramedullary nail and what is the importance of working length?**

   The working length is the length of nail between the most distal point of fixation in the proximal fragment and the most proximal point of fixation in the distal fragment. In other words, it is the unsupported portion of the nail between the bone fragments.

   Torsional stiffness is inversely proportional to working length. Bending stiffness is inversely proportional to the working length to the power of 2.

4. **How does the radius of the nail affect rigidity?**

   For a solid nail, the rigidity/stiffness (to both bending and torsion) is proportional to the radius to the power of 4. For a cannulated nail, rigidity/stiffness is proportional to the radius to the power of 3.

5. **What is the difference between a reamed and an unreamed nail?**

   There are many differences between reamed and unreamed nails.

   Biomechanically, reaming can have several theoretical advantages. It can decrease the working length of the nail in addition to allowing for the insertion of a larger diameter nail. The result of both of these is an increase in the rigidity/stiffness of the construct.

   Unreamed nails theoretically minimise disruption of the endosteal blood supply. However, with reamed nails, there is a six-fold increase in the periosteal blood supply and the direction of the blood flow can reverse from centrifugal to centripetal. Furthermore, there is reconstitution of the endosteal blood supply after 6 weeks. More importantly, the clinical relevance of reaming is such that reamed nails have been shown to have a positive effect on bone union in terms of both rates of union and time to union. This is particularly true in femoral fractures (both open and closed) and closed tibial fractures. The benefits of reaming appear to be less in open fractures of the tibia in clinical trials.

Finally, there is no good evidence to suggest an increased rate of compartment syndrome or pulmonary complications, for example, fat emboli (which occurs with both techniques), when using a reamed nail over an unreamed nail.

6. What are the indications for an external fixator?

I – Temporary fixation
- – Damage control orthopaedics
- – Periarticular fractures: 'Span – scan – plan'
- – Pelvic ring injuries (rarely used these days due to pelvic binders)

II – Definitive treatment
- – Significant soft tissue injuries with associated fractures
- – Paediatric injuries (since they heal faster than adult injuries and the frame is less bothersome to a child)

III – Reconstruction
- – Deformity
- – Infection
- – Non-union
- – Lengthening

7. How does one increase the stiffness of an external fixator?
The most important aspect to an external fixator for increasing stiffness (other than good cortical opposition at the fracture site) is the diameter of pins. The bending stiffness of pins is proportional to the radius of the pins to the power of 4. However, as a rule, no pin should be greater than one-third of the diameter of the bone due to the risk of fracture. Other techniques to increase stiffness include:

- • Pins in different planes (circular > multiplanar > uniplanar)
- • Increasing the number of pins
- • Increasing the space between pins
- • Placement of pins near fracture site
- • Decreasing the distance of rods from bone (this reduces the moment arm)
- • Increasing the diameter of rods
- • Increasing the number of rods

FURTHER READING

Bhandari M, Guyatt GH, Tong D et al. Reamed versus nonreamed intramedullary nailing of lower extremity long bone fractures: A systematic overview and meta-analysis. *J Orthop Trauma.* 2000 Jan;14(1):2–9.

Reichert IL, McCarthy ID, Hughes SP. The acute vascular response to intramedullary reaming. Microsphere estimation of blood flow in the intact ovine tibia. *J Bone Joint Surg Br.* 1995 May;77(3):490–493.

61

NON-UNION

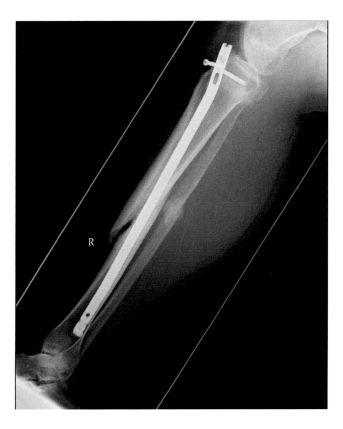

This patient is 1 year down the line following an open fracture of the tibia treated with an intramedullary nail.

1. Describe the radiograph and explain the diagnosis.

This is a lateral radiograph showing a tibial shaft fracture treated with an intramedullary nail. The nail is backing out and the proximal screw is clearly broken. The fracture shows no evidence of healing 12 months post-surgery and therefore this would be described as a non-union.

Treatment with a reamed intramedullary nail for closed fractures has a reported rate of non-union of between 1% and 4%. Following grade 1 open fractures, the rate of non-union remains low, at 2%, but it increases up to 36% for Gustilo and Anderson grade IIIB injuries.

2. What is the definition of a non-union?

A non-union is described as a failure of a fracture to heal within the time frame expected for that specific fracture. The U.S. Food and Drug Administration (FDA) defined non-union as a failure for a fracture to unite by 9 months, with no radiographic progression towards union in the previous 3 months.

3. What are the clinical findings in a non-union?

Clinically, patients may have ongoing pain at the fracture site and, in the lower limb, pain on weight bearing is a classical symptom of non-union. On examination, there may be pain on palpation in addition to movement and crepitus at the fracture site.

In an infected non-union, patients may describe wound problems after surgery such as infected or leaking wounds and may have required antibiotics in the post operative phase. There may be ongoing inflammation at the fracture site in the form of erythema and persistent/night pain may be present, in addition to constitutional symptoms of infection such as sweats, fever, rigors, weight loss and loss of appetite.

4. What is the difference between clinical and radiographic union?

Clinical union is defined as the absence of tenderness or motion at the fracture site with no pain on loading. *Radiographic union* is defined as the presence of visible bridging trabeculae on three out of four cortices on orthogonal radiographs.

5. What are the causes of non-union?

Factors causing non-union can be divided into patient factors, fracture factors or surgical factors.

Patient factors:
- Age (paediatric fractures heal quicker than adult fractures)
- Smoking and excess alcohol
- Drugs (NSAIDs, corticosteroids)
- Medical co-morbidities (diabetes, peripheral vascular disease, malnutrition, anaemia, hypothyroidism, hyperparathyroidism)

Fracture factors:
- Bone involved (femoral shaft take 16 –/+ 4 weeks to unite, whereas a distal radius fracture may heal in under half this time)
- Area of bone involved (diaphyseal fractures generally take longer to heal than metaphyseal fractures). Classically, the distal tibia and proximal pole of the scaphoid are at high risk of non-union
- Fracture type (high-energy fractures, open fractures, comminuted fractures, bone loss, and fractures associated with significant soft tissue damage or periosteal stripping will take longer to heal)
- Infection

Surgical factors:
- Extensive soft tissue damage/periosteal stripping
- Inadequate stability
- Rigid fixation with gapping at the fracture site
- Introduction of infection

6. Do you know of any different types of non-union?

Non-unions can be described as being either hypertrophic or atrophic:

Hypertrophic non-unions are a mechanical problem. They occur when there is a good blood supply but excessive strain at the fracture site prevents progression of the callus to form bone.

Atrophic non-unions are a biological problem. Almost all the patient, fracture, and surgeon factors already discussed can lead to an atrophic non-union. A fracture fixed with rigid fixation but with the fracture fragments distracted will also lack stimulation of callus formation.

7. What are the principles of non-union surgery?

- Eradicate infection
- Excision of interposing tissues
- Restore blood supply
- Stabilisation of bone ends
- Bone graft any fracture gaps

As a general rule, hypertrophic non-unions require increased mechanical stability, usually by compression of the non-union site.

With atrophic non-union, all the principles listed here are required. They need stabilisation and biological enhancement.

8. How would you treat the fracture pictured above?

I would start by investigating for infection with a thorough history (as per Q3) and performing a full set of blood tests including FBC, ESR and CRP. If there was no infection, a non-union of the tibia can be treated very effectively with an exchange nailing with a nail 1–2 millimetres larger in diameter after reaming, and I would send reamings for microscopy, culture and sensitivity to rule out an indolent infection. As above, the increased diameter nail will lead to increased stabilisation of the fracture site and the reaming will deliver autologous bone graft to the fracture site.

The largest cohort of tibial diaphyseal non-unions treated with exchange nailing comes from Edinburgh and, in the aseptic cases, showed a union rate of 75% with a single exchange nailing, rising to 95% with repeat exchange nailing. In the context of infection, exchange nailing had a union rate of 35%, rising only to 61% after a second exchange nailing. Other methods of treatment, such as Ilizarov frames, are therefore indications in infected non-unions.

The radiograph below shows a successful union following exchange nailing.

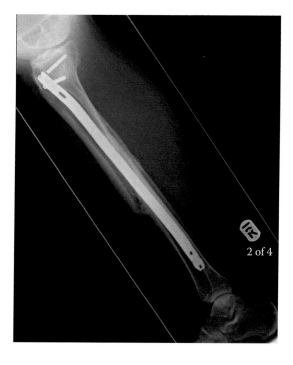

FURTHER READING

Tsang ST, Mills LA, Frantzias J, Baren JP, Keating JF, Simpson AH. Exchange nailing for non-union of diaphyseal fractures of the tibia: Our results and an analysis of the risk factors for failure. *Bone Joint J.* 2016 Apr;98-B(4):534–541.

62

NON-ACCIDENTAL INJURY

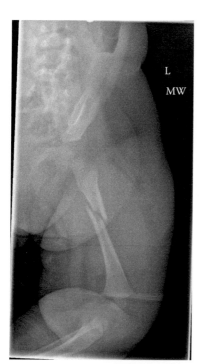
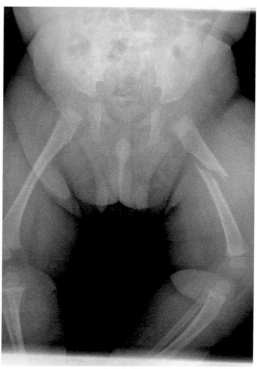

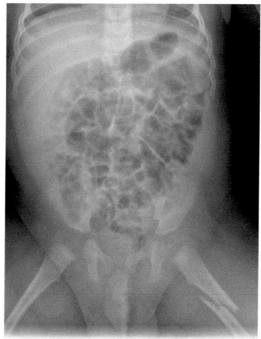

You are the orthopaedic registrar on call. You are called to the emergency department to see a 4-month-old child with a displaced midshaft diaphyseal femoral fracture who has been brought to hospital by his mother because he is distressed and inconsolable. The given history is that he may have rolled off the bed onto the floor 2 days previously.

1. **How would you manage this patient and family in the emergency department?**
   I would take the history from the mother, examine the child and record both carefully. There are a number of concerning features about this presentation. A femoral fracture in a non-ambulatory child would alert me to the possibility of a non-accidental injury. The delay in presentation is also concerning. I would also look to corroborate the history from any other family members attending.

   I would be looking for any other sign of injury to the child, evidence of neglect and a normal interaction between mother and child. I would also consider the possibility of a skeletal dysplasia as a cause of bone fragility and would ask the mother about any suggestive family history. I would consult with the senior emergency department doctor and my consultant. I would admit the child for analgesia and fracture management. I would treat this child with a Pavlik harness for 4 weeks in the expectation that this would stabilise the fracture, allow it to heal and there would be subsequent remodelling. In my hospital, I would contact the on-call paediatrician responsible for child protection who would take the lead in this regard and coordinate any investigation including the involvement of social services and arranging further investigations such as a skeletal survey.

2. **What features in a presentation or injury might make you worry about non-accidental injury?**
   Characteristic injuries seen in non-accidental injury are skull fractures, rib fractures, femoral fractures in non-ambulatory children (younger than 18 months), humeral fractures and several co-existing or multiple fractures which may be of different ages. These are increasingly sensitive when seen in combination.

   Other features which should alert the clinician might include a delay in presentation, presentation out of hours and evidence of neglect. Some studies have suggested that metaphyseal corner fractures or certain bruising patterns might indicate non-accidental injury. The evidence for this is less clear. Nevertheless, where there is concern, most hospitals have a clear policy as to how concerns should be raised. I would discuss my concerns with my consultant on call and with the paediatrician on call for child protection.

3. **Are you aware of any relevant literature in this area?**
   Worlock P, Stower M, Barbor P. Patterns of fractures in accidental and non-accidental injury in children: A comparative study. *Br Med J (Clin Res Ed)*. 1986 Jul 12;293(6539):100–102.

   A cohort study undertaken over 6 years comparing fracture patterns in children sustained as non-accidental injuries with those where abuse/NAI had been excluded. Multiple fractures, bruising to the head and neck, spiral humeral fractures and rib fractures were associated with NAI. Metaphyseal 'chip' fractures were uncommon.

Kemp AM, Dunstan F, Harrison S, Morris S, Mann M, Rolfe K, Datta S, Thomas DP, Sibert JR, Maguire S. Patterns of skeletal fractures in child abuse: Systematic review. *BMJ*. 2008 Oct 2;337:a1518. doi: 10.1136/bmj.a1518.

A systematic review of 32 papers/studies examining fracture patterns in non-accidental injury. No single fracture type or pattern is pathognomic for non-accidental injury; however, multiple fractures are commonly seen in NAI and fractures to the ribs, femur or humerus were also associated with NAI in the absence of major trauma.

63

OSTEOPOROSIS

You review a 67-year-old woman in the fracture clinic. She has had a distal radius fracture after a fall. The fracture is in a good position and you have agreed that she will be treated in a cast. She asks if she should be taking something for 'weak bones'.

1. **What advice would you offer?**

    I would take a targeted history from this woman, looking to identify the energy of her injury: It appears to be a low-energy fall. I would also explore any potential risk factors for osteoporosis or osteopenia. Her fixed risk factors include age, sex, family history of osteoporosis and her ethnicity. Modifiable risk factors include current or previous frequent use of steroids, premature menopause or ovarian failure as well as alcohol and cigarette use. In a female patient over the age 65 years or a man over the age of 75 years with one or more of these risk factors, the risk of osteoporosis and resulting fragility fractures is increased and bone protection may be appropriate.

    I would suggest that the patient is investigated with a bone mineral density scan. In my hospital, patients are referred for this routinely based on screening of fracture clinic referrals and the results are passed to the general practitioner who is able to decide on appropriate management or referral with the patient.

2. **What are the key outputs from a DEXA scan and how would you interpret these figures?**

    The DEXA scan produces a measure of bone mineral density (BMD) expressed as two figures, the T-score and the Z-score. Both are expressed in units of standard deviation. The T-score compares the patient bone mineral density to that of a healthy 30 year old of the same sex and ethnicity. This is the most important score. The Z-score is an age-matched score comparison. It allows comparison of bone mass with patients of the same age, sex, race, height and weight.

    If the T-score is greater than –1 SD, this is normal. Osteopenia is diagnosed when the T-score is between –1 and –2.5 SD. Osteoporosis is diagnosed with a T-score of –2.5 SD or below. A Z-score of –2 SD or below indicates a lower bone mineral density than expected for a healthy adult of the same age.

    While these investigations give a measure of bone mineral density, the fracture risk for a patient is also affected by factors such as a history of falls or previous fracture. These should be considered with the bone mineral density results when determining if bone protection is appropriate. The World Health Organisation Fracture Risk Assessment Tool (FRAX) is one way of making this assessment.

    Local practice in my hospital is based on NICE guidance. Post-menopausal women and men over the age of 50 with a T-score of –2.5 or less are, after appropriate counselling, recommended to be prescribed a bisphosphonate. Where dietary calcium intake is adequate, supplementary vitamin D is recommended if sunlight exposure is limited. Hormone replacement therapy is considered for women who suffer premature menopause.

3. **Can you tell me about the agents used for the treatment of osteoporosis and explain how these act?**

There is formal NICE guidance for this. All patients diagnosed with osteoporosis or who are at risk of fragility fracture should receive general lifestyle advice.

- Patients are prescribed vitamin D (800 IU) and calcium (1500 mg) supplements daily.
- Bisphosphonates: These are the most common pharmacologic agents used. They inhibit osteoclast activity by attaching to the ruffled border of the osteoclast and so reduce bone resorption. There are risks associated with the use of bisphosphonates; atypical proximal femoral fractures and osteonecrosis of the jaw have been described. Both are rare but the risk of femoral fracture particularly means that it is recommended that bisphosphonate treatment should be reviewed with a repeat fracture risk assessment after 5 years of treatment. Patients who remain at high fracture risk or who have very low BMD are recommended to continue lifelong treatment. Where the fracture risk has improved or a repeat bone scan shows a T-score at or close to –2.5 then a 'treatment holiday' of 1–2 years may be advised in order to reduce the risk of proximal femoral fracture.
- Strontium ranelate is a second-line drug and acts by activating osteoblasts and encouraging bone production.
- Oestrogen receptor modulators such as Raloxifene attach to oestrogen receptors in bone and encourage bone formation.

FURTHER READING

Osteoporosis: Assessing the risk of fragility fracture. Nice Guidelines [CG146]. August 2012. Accessed from https://www.nice.org.uk/guidance/cg146/chapter/1-Guidance.

SECTION IV
SURGICAL APPROACHES

64

DELTOPECTORAL APPROACH

1. **What are the indications for the deltopectoral approach?**
   The deltopectoral approach affords excellent anterior access to the glenohumoral joint and is used for:

   - Proximal humerus ORIF
   - Arthroplasty
   - Open washout septic glenohumeral joint
   - Open reduction of irreducible anterior dislocations

2. **What is the internervous plane utilised by this approach?**
   Deltoid (axillary nerve) laterally
   Pectoralis major (medial and lateral pectoral nerves) medially

3. **How would you position the patient?**
   I would utilise the beach chair position. This would include sitting the patient up at 45 degrees, placing two pillows under the knees, and formal head support/head ring reinforced with a crepe bandage.

4. **Where would you make your incision?**
   An incision is made in the line of the deltopectoral groove, from the coracoid process, along the deltopectoral groove to the lateral arm.

5. **Talk me through the superficial dissection.**
   After making my skin incision (as above) I would achieve haemostasis due to the bleeding that can occur from superficial skin vessels and identify the deltopectoral fascia. The cephalic vein lies in a layer of fat and is used to identify the interval between the deltoid and pec major. I would retract the cephalic vein (usually laterally as the tributaries come from the lateral side) and divide the deltopectoral fascia of the arm.

6. **What about the deep dissection?**

   - Identify the coracoid process.
   - Divide the clavipectoral fascia from the coracoid process down along the lateral border of conjoint tendon.
   - Retract conjoint tendon medially, with care taken to avoid overzealous retraction and damage to the musculocutaneous nerve, and retract the deltoid laterally.
   - This will allow for identification of the subscapularis tendon. Externally rotate the arm to put the subscapularis under tension.
   - Place stay sutures in the lateral part of the subscapularis tendon and divide in tendinous portion and take off capsule under tension.
   - Perform a vertical capsulotomy to enter the joint.

7. What are the dangers of this approach?

- Musculocutaneous nerve: This enters the coracobrachialis muscle as close as 2.5 cm distal to the tip of the coracoid. Vigorous retraction can lead to damage to this nerve.
- Axillary nerve: This is at risk during the incision in the subscapularis tendon, where it lies just distal to the tendon as it wraps around the humerus from lateral to medial.
- Cephalic vein: This can cause bleeding if damaged intraoperatively, and will increase surgical oedema if damaged and ligated.

8. How would you extend this approach?

This can be extended distally into an anterior (brachialis splitting) approach to the humerus (see Chapter 65).

65

ANTERIOR APPROACH TO HUMERUS

1. **What are the indications for the anterior (brachialis splitting) approach to the humerus?**
   The main indication is for the ORIF of proximal and middle third diaphyseal humerus fractures. It is limited in that it cannot be extended distally but it can be extended proximally using the deltopectoral interval.

   Other indications include humeral osteotomies and tumour biopsies/resections.

2. **What is the internervous plane utilised by this approach?**
   The anterior approach utilises the internervous plane between the medial two-thirds of brachialis (supplied by the musculocutaneous nerve) and the lateral one-third of brachialis (supplied by the radial nerve). The radial nerve fibres supplying brachialis are largely proprioceptive in nature.

3. **How would you position the patient?**
   Supine with the arm abducted to 60 degrees on an arm board.

4. **Where would you base your incision?**
   I would make a longitudinal incision over the lateral border of the biceps, starting about 15 cm proximal to the elbow crease and ending approximately 5 cm proximal to it.

5. **Talk me through the superficial dissection.**
   After making my skin incision (as above) I would identify and retract the cephalic vein and divide the deep fascia of the arm in line with the incision to identify the lateral border of the biceps.

6. **What about the deep dissection?**
   I would identify the muscular interval between the biceps and brachialis and develop this interval by retracting the biceps medially to reveal the whole of brachialis which overlies the humeral shaft. I would identify the musculocutaneous nerve at this stage and avoid it during splitting of brachialis.

   To expose the humeral shaft, I would split the fibres of brachialis (two thirds medial/one third lateral) and expose the periosteum of the anterior humeral shaft. I would incise the periosteum and strip brachialis off the bone, trying to preserve as much soft tissue attachment as possible.

7. **What are the dangers of this approach?**
   The radial nerve. This can be damaged with overzealous stripping of muscle from bone, and care must be taken to remain in a subperiosteal plane without dissecting too far posteriorly. It may also be injured by drills or screws placed from anterior to posterior in the mid-diaphysis of the humerus.

   In the distal third of the arm, the radial nerve has pierced the lateral inter-muscular septum and lies in the anterior compartment between brachialis and

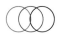

brachioradialis. When brachialis is split, leaving a lateral cuff of muscle, this acts to protect the radial nerve from retractors.

Musculocutaneous nerve: This overlies brachialis and must be identified prior to splitting brachialis. It then continues down the arm and becomes the lateral cutaneous nerve of the forearm.

8. How would you extend this approach?

This approach can only be extended proximally. This would utilise the deltopectoral approach to the proximal humerus (see separate station in Chapter 7).

66

ANTEROLATERAL APPROACH TO HUMERUS

1. **What are the indications for the anterolateral approach to the humerus?**
   The main indication is for the ORIF of middle-third and distal-third diaphyseal humerus fractures. Unlike the anterior approach, it can be extended both proximally and distally.

   Other indications include exploration of the radial nerve, humeral osteotomies and tumour biopsies/resections.

2. **What is the internervous plane utilised by this approach?**
   There is no true internervous plane. This approach uses an intermuscular plane as both the lateral third of brachialis and brachioradialis muscles are supplied by the radial nerve.

3. **How would you position the patient?**
   Supine with the arm abducted to 60 degrees on an arm board.

4. **Where would you base your incision?**
   I would make a curved longitudinal incision over the lateral border of the biceps, starting about 10 cm proximal to the elbow crease and ending just proximal to it.

5. **Talk me through the superficial dissection.**
   After making my skin incision (as above) I would identify and retract the cephalic vein and divide the deep fascia of the arm in line with the incision to identify the lateral border of the biceps.

   The lateral cutaneous nerve of forearm (LCNF) crosses from medial to lateral under the fascia. Approximately 5 cm proximal to the elbow crease, it emerges from between the biceps and brachialis as the continuation of the musculocutaneous nerve. It should be retracted with the biceps.

6. **What about the deep dissection?**
   Retract biceps medially along with the LCNF to identify the interval between brachioradialis and brachialis. Incise the deep fascia in line with the intermuscular septum between brachioradialis and brachialis and develop the intermuscular plane to find the radial nerve. The radial nerve is most readily identified distally between these two muscles. Mobilise and protect the nerve and trace it back up the lateral humerus to where it pierces the lateral intermuscular septum. Brachialis is then stripped with a periosteal elevator and retracted medially to expose the anterior shaft of the distal humerus.

7. **What are the dangers of this approach?**
   Radial nerve
   Lateral cutaneous nerve of forearm

8. How would you extend this approach?

This extensile approach can be extended proximally or distally.

Proximally, the plane between brachialis medially and the lateral head of the triceps posterolaterally can be utilised. Posterior dissection may injure the radial nerve in the spiral groove and therefore any dissection should be subperiosteal.

Distally, the anterolateral approach can be extended into the anterior approach to the elbow/proximal forearm by developing the same internervous plane at the elbow and, in the proximal forearm, between brachioradialis (radial nerve) and pronator teres (median nerve).

9. When would you use the anterolateral approach over the anterior approach?

The anterior approach cannot be extended distally, nor does it allow for exploration of the radial nerve. Therefore, the anterolateral approach is used over the anterior approach where there is any requirement for distal extension down the humeral shaft or the radial nerve requires exploration.

67

POSTERIOR APPROACH
TO DISTAL HUMERUS

1. **What are the indications for the posterior approach to the humerus?**
   The main indication is for ORIF of the middle third and distal third humerus fractures including intra-articular distal humerus fractures as well as arthroplasty of the elbow joint.

2. **What is the internervous plane utilised by this approach?**
   There is no true internervous plane. This approach involves separating the three heads of triceps, all of which are supplied by the radial nerve. The medial head, in the deepest part of the dissection, has a dual innervation from the radial and ulnar nerves. Therefore, splitting the medial head longitudinally avoids denervation of either half. The other two heads receive their nerve supply near their origins and therefore longitudinal splitting of these muscles results in no denervation either.

3. **How would you position the patient?**
   The patient is positioned in the lateral position with the affected side uppermost. The arm is brought out in front of the patient and placed over a bolster. A very high arm tourniquet is paramount such that it does not interfere with the sterile surgical field.

4. **Where would you base your incision?**
   The skin incision is made in the mid-line of the posterior aspect of the arm, centred over the fracture site in the context of trauma.

5. **Talk me through the superficial dissection.**
   After making my skin incision, I would incise the deep fascia of the arm in line with the skin incision. The superficial layer of triceps contains the lateral head and the long head. The interval between these two muscles is developed and the lateral head is retracted laterally; the long head, medially.

6. **What about the deep dissection?**
   The medial head lies deep to the other two heads. The radial nerve runs in the spiral groove just proximal to the medial head of triceps. To expose the posterior humeral shaft, the medial head is incised in its mid-line down to the periosteum. Remaining in the subperiosteal plane avoids damage to the ulnar nerve which pierces the medial intermuscular septum to enter the posterior compartment of the arm approximately 8 cm proximal to the medial epicondyle.

7. **What are the dangers of this approach?**

   - Radial nerve: It crosses the posterior aspect of humerus approximately 20 cm proximal to the medial epicondyle and 15 cm proximal to the lateral epicondyle. Dissection down to the bone in the proximal two-thirds of the humerus should never take place until the nerve has been identified.

- Profunda brachii: This runs with the radial nerve in the spiral groove.
- Ulnar nerve: As above.

8. How would you extend this approach?

This approach can be extended distally to address intra-articular fractures. The skin incision is extended distally over the olecranon and an olecranon osteotomy is made.

This approach cannot be extended proximally due to the radial nerve in the spiral groove and the deltoid muscle crossing the operative field.

68

ANTERIOR/VOLAR (HENRY'S) APPROACH TO THE FOREARM

1. What are the indications for a volar approach to the forearm?

- ORIF of fractures
- Bone grafting and fixation of non-unions
- Osteotomies
- Biopsy and treatment of bone tumours
- Anterior exposure of bicipital tuberosity
- Compartment syndrome of the forearm

2. What is the internervous plane utilised by this approach?
The internervous planes are the same (radial nerve laterally and median nerve medially) throughout the forearm, but the muscles encountered are different proximally and distally:

Proximally, I would retract brachioradialis (radial nerve) laterally and pronator teres (median nerve) medially
Distally, the brachioradialis (radial nerve) is taken laterally and flexor carpi radialis (medial nerve) medially

3. How would you position the patient?
I would position the patient supine with an arm table attachment and an upper arm tourniquet. I wouldn't exsanguinate the arm in order to keep the veins engorged. This assists with identification of the venae comitantes of the radial artery.

4. Where would you base your incision?
The approach utilises an incision, which starts at the elbow flexor crease, medial to mobile wad, extending to the styloid process of the radius distally.

5. Talk me through the superficial dissection.
I would extend the incision down through fat, taking care not to damage the cephalic vein, then identify the deep fascia. I would incise the deep fascia of the forearm in line with the skin incision. I would then identify the ulnar border of brachioradialis and develop the plane between it and flexor carpi radialis (FCR) distally and pronator teres proximally. Brachioradialis is the retracted laterally and pronator teres/FCR is taken medially. It may be necessary to ligate/coagulate the leash of Henry (recurrent branches of the radial artery) to mobilise the brachioradialis laterally and the radial artery medially. The superficial radial nerve runs on the underside of brachioradialis and is retracted laterally with the muscle.

6. Can you describe the deep dissection?

Usually only a portion of the approach is required and the deep dissection can be split into thirds: proximal, middle, distal. The arm should be supinated, pronated, supinated, respectively depending on the level of the fracture.

Proximal Third (forearm supinated)

The biceps insertion into the bicipital tuberosity of the radius is identified.

The radial artery is medial to the biceps tendon at this level, therefore the plane between biceps tendon and brachioradialis (laterally) is developed.

The proximal third of the radius is covered by the supinator, through which the posterior interosseus nerve (PIN) travels en route to the posterior compartment of the forearm.

Supination displaces the PIN from the surgical field and exposes the insertion of the supinator onto the anterior portion of the proximal radius. (Supination of the forearm will not have this effect when there is a radial shaft fracture, but can be achieved with bone reduction forceps.)

The supinator is incised in line with the radius and stripped subperiosteally in a radial direction, further displacing the PIN from the surgical field. Any retraction is performed carefully, as the PIN is at risk of a neurapraxia, which can take many months to recover. (NB: Never place retractors on the posterior surface of the radial neck, as these may compress the PIN, which comes into direct contact with this area in some patients.)

Middle Third (forearm pronated)

The middle third of the radial shaft is covered by pronator teres (PT) and flexor digitorum superficialis (FDS) muscles.

The arm is then pronated to expose the insertion of PT onto the lateral radial shaft.

The insertion is detached and the muscle is stripped off in an ulnar direction, which also detaches the origin of FDS.

Distal Third (forearm supinated)

The traditional Henry's approach is radial to the radial artery, between brachioradialis and the radial artery.

Two muscles arise from the anterior distal third of the radius: Pronator quadratus (PQ) and flexor pollicis longus (both innervated by the anterior interosseus nerve).

The radial portion of PQ is incised and peeled off the distal radius in an ulnar direction with subperiosteal dissection.

My preferred approach in this region is the modified Henry's approach to the distal radius through the bed of FCR. The sheath of FCR is incised and the tendon freed, before retracting this in an ulnar direction to protect the median nerve (radial artery is retracted radially) and going through the bed of FCR.

The sheath over FPL is incised and FPL is retracted ulnarly by sweeping this with a finger to reveal pronator quadratus (PQ).

To expose the distal radius, the radial portion of PQ is incised and peeled off the distal radius in an ulnar direction with subperiosteal dissection.

7. What are the dangers of this approach?

Superficial radial nerve: This lies on the underside of brachioradialis and can be damaged with vigorous retraction.

Radial artery: This lies on the ulnar side of brachioradialis and can be damaged if not identified. Use of a tourniquet without exsanguination can allow for easier identification of the venae comitantes.

PIN: This travels through the body of the supinator and can be damaged when exposing the proximal third of the radial shaft. Retractors placed on the posterior surface of the radial neck may compress the PIN, which comes into direct contact with this area in some patients.

Cephalic vein: This commences in the anatomical snuffbox and runs from here, across the volar aspect of the forearm to the antecubital fossa. It is at risk in the superficial dissection of this approach, particularly in the proximal third.

8. How may this approach be extended?

This approach can be extended proximally across the elbow into an anterolateral approach to the arm (see Chapter 67). Distally, the approach can be extended to allow for carpal tunnel decompression, for example, high-energy distal radius fractures with progressive median nerve symptoms. My preferred approach would be to perform a separate incision over the carpal tunnel to avoid crossing the path of the palmar cutaneous and recurrent motor branch of the median nerve.

69

KOCHER'S AND KAPLAN'S APPROACHES

1. **What are the indications for the Kocher's approach to the humerus?**
   Excision/ORIF/replacement of radial head
   Terrible triad ORIF

2. **What is the internervous plane utilised by this approach?**
   This plane is between anconeus (radial nerve) and extensor carpi ulnaris (posterior interosseus nerve). This approach does not utilise a true internervous plane as the posterior interosseus nerve (PIN) is itself a branch of the radial nerve.

3. **How would you position the patient?**
   Supine with the upper limb on an arm board. The forearm should be pronated to remove the PIN from the surgical field as it passes through the supinator.

4. **Where would you base your incision?**
   Incise the skin obliquely from a point 1 cm proximal to the lateral epicondyle, extending distally to a point 6 cm distal to the tip of the olecranon.

   For surgical treatment of a terrible triad injury, I would utilise a midline posterior skin incision – the utility approach to the elbow – through skin, fat and fascia, at which point large fasciocutaneous flaps can be raised on both sides. The elbow has an excellent blood supply and flap viability is rarely problematic. The Kocher's interval would then be utilised, and this also gives the option of a medial approach to the elbow through the bed of the ulnar nerve if required.

5. **Talk me through the dissection.**
   Incise the superficial fascia in line with the skin incision.

   To find the interval between anconeus and ECU, look distally (as they share a common aponeurosis proximally) for a thin strip of fat and incise the aponeurosis in this line lifting the anconeus flap anteriorly and the ECU flap posteriorly. This reveals the capsule of the elbow joint.

   Incise the capsule in line with the incision to reveal the capitellum, the radial head and the annular ligament. The PIN is at risk here if the arm is not fully pronated.

6. **What are the dangers of this approach?**
   Radial nerve: Can be damaged if the capsule is opened too far anterior.
   PIN: Can be injured if the forearm is not pronated or, given its proximity to the radial neck, it may be injured if retractors are placed around this. Staying proximal to the annular ligament will prevent injury to the PIN and is the reason why this approach cannot be extended distally.

7. How does Kaplan's interval differ from Kocher's interval?

Kaplan's interval utilises an internervous plane between the extensor carpi radialis brevis (radial nerve) and extensor digitorum communis (PIN). This is the same interval utilised by the Thompson (dorsal) approach to the radius in the proximal third of the forearm. There is a higher risk of PIN injury utilising this approach and therefore many surgeons prefer the Kocher's interval for access to the radial head and lateral side of the elbow.

70

SMITH–PETERSEN APPROACH

1. **What are the indications for the anterior approach to the hip?**
   This approach is predominantly used for irrigation and debridement of a septic arthritis of a native hip, or for reduction of displaced intracapsular hip fractures in the young.

   Other uses for this approach include irreducible anterior dislocations of the hip, paediatric pelvic osteotomies, open reduction of DDH, arthrodesis and arthroplasty of the hip and tumour excision.

2. **What is the internervous plane utilised by this approach?**
   The internervous plane is between the femoral nerve and the superior gluteal nerve. Superficially, the plane is between sartorius (femoral nerve) medially and tensor fascia latae (superior gluteal nerve) laterally. The deep dissection utilises the internervous plane between rectus femoris (femoral nerve) medially and gluteus medius (superior gluteal nerve) laterally.

3. **How would you position the patient?**
   Supine. The leg would be externally rotated initially to stretch the sartorius muscle to make it more prominent and also to stretch the capsule when making the capsulotomy.

4. **Where would you base your skin incision?**
   In an adult, I would base the incision along the anterior half of the iliac crest to the anterior superior iliac spine (ASIS). I would then curve the incision down so that it runs vertically for approximately 10 cm, heading towards the lateral side of the patella. The incision can start at the ASIS for indications such as washout of a native hip and reduction of a displaced intracapsular hip fracture. In a child, for washout of a septic hip joint, I would place a curvilinear skin incision in the groin crease.

5. **Can you describe the superficial dissection?**
   Externally rotate the leg to stretch the sartorius muscle.

   Blunt dissection through the subcutaneous fat will avoid damage to the lateral cutaneous nerve of the thigh, which pierces the deep fascia of the thigh near this intermuscular interval between sartorius and tensor fascia latae (TFL).

   Identify the internervous interval (which is easiest to palpate 2 to 3 inches below the ASIS) between sartorius medially and TFL laterally.

   Incise the deep fascia over the medial portion TFL to protect the lateral cutaneous nerve of the thigh, which usually lies just under the fascia of sartorius.

   Retract the sartorius medially along with the nerve and the tensor fascia latae laterally and identify the ascending branch of the lateral circumflex femoral artery (which crosses the gap between sartorius and TFL): This must be ligated or coagulated.

6. What about the deep dissection?

Develop plane between rectus femoris (femoral nerve) medially and gluteus medius (superior gluteal nerve) laterally.

If you are struggling for exposure, the origins of rectus femoris (straight head from the ASIS and reflected head from the superior lip of the acetabulum) can be detached to retract rectus femoris further medially, thus exposing the capsule.

Adduct and fully externally rotate the leg to put the capsule on stretch, then define the capsule with blunt dissection. Incise the hip joint capsule either longitudinally or with a T-shaped capsulotomy, depending on the extent of exposure required.

7. What are the dangers of this approach?

Lateral cutaneous nerve of the thigh:

- Reaches thigh by passing under inguinal ligament, generally 1 cm medial to the ASIS.
- The course is variable and it is most commonly seen when incising fascia between the sartorius and TFL.
- Injury may lead to painful neuroma or reduced sensation on the lateral aspect of thigh.

Ascending branch of lateral femoral circumflex artery:

- Found proximally in the internervous plane between the tensor fascia latae and sartorius.
- Must be ligated or coagulated to prevent brisk bleeding from this large vessel.

8. How can this approach be extended?

The approach can be extended proximally along the iliac crest to expose bone for harvesting bone graft.

Distally, the skin incision can be extended down the anterolateral aspect of the thigh and through the fascia lata. The interval between rectus femoris and vastus lateralis can be utilised to gain access to the entire femoral shaft.

71

ILIOINGUINAL APPROACH

1. **What are the indications for the ilioinguinal approach?**
   Operative management of acetabular fractures.

   The ilioinguinal approach allows for excellent access to the front of the pelvis as well as visualisation of a large area of its internal surface from the sacroiliac joint to the pubic symphysis. It can be used for virtually all fractures of the anterior column and anterior wall. The majority of both column fractures can also be treated with this approach.

   Articular reductions are done indirectly. They are based on meticulous restoration of extra-articular anatomy, since the joint cannot be directly visualised with this approach. (NB: There is no true internervous plane for this approach – the dissection consists of lifting off muscular, nervous and vascular structures from the inner wall of the pelvis.)

2. **How would you position the patient?**
   I would position the patient supine on a radiolucent pelvic surgery table. I would place a sandbag under the ipsilateral buttock and insert a urinary catheter to empty the bladder. I would check that the C-arm image intensifier can be positioned to obtain satisfactory obturator and iliac oblique views as well as inlet and outlet views of the pelvis.

3. **Describe how you would perform the skin incision.**
   I would make a curved incision from the iliac crest, starting approximately 5 cm superior to the anterior superior iliac spine (ASIS), extending medially to the pubic symphysis.

4. **Describe how you would perform the superficial dissection.**
   After dissecting down through fat, the aponeurosis of the external oblique muscle is exposed. Caution is required in the lateral portion of the wound as the lateral cutaneous nerve may be encountered due to its variable anatomy. The aponeurosis is divided in the line of its fibres from 1 cm above the superficial inguinal ring to the anterior superior iliac spine to deroof the inguinal canal. This exposes the spermatic cord (in men) or round ligament (in women) which can be mobilised and protected by a sling. The ilioinguinal nerve accompanies the spermatic cord/round ligament in the inguinal canal and this should also be identified and protected.

   Medially, I would extend my dissection by dividing the anterior part of the rectus sheath to expose the rectus abdominis muscle.

   Laterally, I would incise the periosteum along the iliac crest, releasing the abdominal and iliacus muscle insertions from the ilium and I would subperiosteally elevate the iliacus from the internal iliac fossa to the SI joint and pelvic brim (the superior edge of the pelvic inlet). I would then pack the internal iliac fossa for haemostasis.

5. **Describe how you would perform the deep dissection.**
   Deep dissection is performed to allow access and surgery performed through three 'operative windows'. Not all of these will necessarily be required, so the deep dissection is tailored to the injury pattern. These operative windows are the lateral, middle and medial windows.

Medial Window

I would divide the rectus abdominal muscle transversely 1 cm proximal to its insertion into the symphysis pubis and utilise blunt dissection to develop the plane between the back of the pubic symphysis and the bladder (Cave of Retzius/ retropubic space), followed by protection of the bladder with a malleable retractor.

I would then cut through the fibres of the internal oblique and transversus abdominus muscles that form the posterior wall of the inguinal canal medially.

Caution: The Corona mortis (a retropubic vascular communication between the external iliac and obturator arteries) must be ligated if this anatomical variant is present.

Middle Window

I would divide the transversus abdominus and internal oblique muscles that arise from the lateral half of the inguinal ligament. I would then gently push the peritoneum upwards to reveal the femoral vessels, the femoral nerve and the tendon of iliopsoas, which I would isolate with slings.

The iliopectineal fascia separates the neural and vascular compartments and blocks access to the true pelvis from the internal iliac fossa. The fascia is delineated by careful retraction of the femoral vessels medially and the femoral nerve and iliopsoas laterally. It is then divided distally, under direct visualisation, down to the pubic root. The iliopsoas is then retracted laterally, exposing the fascial attachment to the pelvic brim which can be divided safely.

Once the iliopectineal fascia has been released, the true pelvis can be entered from the internal iliac fossa.

Dissection around the iliac vessels should be minimised. This limits risk of vascular injury and also preserves the path of the primary lymphatic trunk to the lower extremity which passes medial to the vein.

Caution:

- The lateral cutaneous nerve of the thigh is usually encountered just deep to the conjoint tendon (of the internal oblique and the transversus abdominis), approximately 1–2 cm medial to the anterior superior iliac spine. This nerve can usually be preserved if it is mobilised as it exits the abdominal wall and enters the fascia of the thigh.
- Inferior epigastric artery crosses the posterior wall of the canal at the medial edge of the deep inguinal ring.

Lateral Window

This is developed by releasing the iliacus muscle from the inner surface of the pelvis as described previously.

Summary

Window	Boundaries	Access to
Lateral	Lateral to the iliopsoas tendon and femoral nerve	The entire internal iliac fossa from the SI joint posteriorly to the iliopectineal eminence anteriorly
Middle	Between the iliopsoas tendon/ femoral nerve laterally and the femoral vessels medially	Pelvic brim, quadrilateral plate, and a portion of the superior ramus
Medial	Medial to the femoral vessels	Superior pubic ramus and pubic symphysis

6. What structures are at risk during this approach?

Lateral cutaneous nerve of the thigh: This will appear in the lateral edge of your incision, medial to the ASIS. It generally lies 1 cm medial but can be extremely variable.

Femoral vessels: These are at risk throughout the deep dissection and careful and judicious retraction must be placed on these at all times to prevent injury or provoke thrombus formation.

Ilioinguinal nerve: This accompanies the spermatic cord/round ligament in the inguinal canal and this should be identified and protected.

72

POSTEROLATERAL APPROACH TO ANKLE

1. **What are the indications for the posterolateral approach to the ankle?**
   This approach is generally used for pilon fractures and ankle fracture surgery, especially to access the posterior malleolus fracture fragment where there is a large, displaced posterior malleolus fracture that cannot be reduced by closed means or held reliably from anterior to posterior. A long oblique fracture which may tend to displace due to shear forces may benefit from a posterior malleolus buttress plate. The fibula can often be plated through the same incision if required.

2. **What is the internervous plane utilised by this approach?**
   This internervous plane is between the peroneal tendons laterally (superficial peroneal nerve) and the flexor hallucis longus (FHL) medially (tibial nerve).

3. **How would you position the patient?**
   The patient can be placed prone or lateral for this approach. My preference is to place the patient in the lateral position, injured side uppermost.

4. **Where would you base your incisions and what structures must be avoided?**
   I would be vigilant to ensure to leave an adequate skin bridge of 7 centimetres or more between the two incisions to reduce the risk of tissue necrosis affecting the skin bridge.

5. **Talk me through the dissection.**
   I would use blunt dissection in the superficial fat. The sural nerve runs with the short saphenous vein at this level and should be preserved where possible and protected to prevent a painful neuroma. A plane is then developed between the peroneal tendons laterally and the Achilles tendon medially in order to reveal the FHL muscle belly, which is low-lying and often extends to the level of the ankle joint, hence the term 'beef to the heel' used to describe it.

   To access the posterior malleolus, a longitudinal incision is made through the lateral fibres of the FHL as they arise from the fibula. The FHL is then retracted medially to reveal the periosteum overlying the posterior malleolus.

   To access the fibula through this approach, the peroneal tendons are retracted medially, giving excellent access to the posterior distal fibula.

6. **How is the sural nerve formed and what does it supply?**
   The sural nerve is formed by branches of the tibial nerve (medial sural cutaneous nerve) and the common peroneal nerve (lateral sural cutaneous nerve) and crosses from medial to lateral, crossing the lateral border of the Achilles tendon approximately 10 cm proximal to its insertion. The sural nerve is purely sensory: It supplies the lateral aspect of the foot.

7. **What are the dangers of this approach?**
   Short saphenous vein and sural nerve as above.

73

LEG FASCIOTOMY (TWO-INCISION/ FOUR-COMPARTMENT FASCIOTOMY)

1. **What are the most common causes implicated in the development of compartment syndrome?**

   - Tibial diaphyseal fracture
   - Soft tissue injury, including crush injuries
   - Distal radius fracture (particularly young men with high-energy injuries)
   - Diaphyseal forearm fracture
   - Diaphyseal femoral fracture
   - Tibial plateau fracture
   - Other causes include burns, revascularisation, extravasation of IV fluid and exercise

2. **How would you position the patient to perform a leg fasciotomy?**
   I would position the patient supine with a thigh tourniquet applied but not inflated. I would place a sandbag under the ipsilateral buttock to 'roll the lower limb in' and to allow access to the lateral aspect of the leg. Following completion of the lateral fasciotomy I would ask the theatre floor staff to remove the sandbag so that the lower limb 'rolls out' to allow access for the medial fasciotomy.

3. **Where would you base your incisions and what structures must be avoided?**
   I would utilise a two-incision approach. The lateral incision will be used to decompress the anterior and lateral compartments. This is based 3–4 cm lateral to the anterior tibial border, midway between the tibia and the fibula.

   The medial incision will be used to decompress the superficial and deep posterior compartments. This is based 1–2 cm posterior to the medial tibial border. The medial incision must be anterior to the posterior tibial artery in order to avoid injuring the 10-cm perforator on the medial side (this is usually the largest and most reliable for distally based fasciocutaneous flaps). There are 5/10/15 cm perforators on the medial side, measured at distances from the medial malleolus, although these are variable. The medial incision is also based anterior to avoid the saphenous vein and nerve.

   One must be vigilant and ensure they leave a satisfactory skin bridge (>7 cm) between the two incisions to avoid potential necrosis of the skin bridge.

4. **Talk me through the superficial and deep dissection.**

   Lateral
   > Blunt dissection through fat distally to identify the superficial peroneal nerve (SPN) as it pierces the deep fascia (typically 10–15 cm proximal to the lateral malleolus).
   > Incise the deep fascia with a scalpel at the midpoint overlying the anterior compartment, then extend proximally and distally with scissors with a closed tip.
   > Then incise the deep fascia overlying the lateral compartment in a similar fashion.

Medial

Blunt dissection through the fat to protect the long saphenous vein and saphenous nerve. Incise the deep fascia anterior to these as above with a scalpel and then closed-tip scissors to open the superficial posterior compartment.

To decompress the deep posterior compartment from the medial side, one must incise the fascia overlying FDL. Distally, this is superficial and can be incised directly.

Proximally, however, soleus is blocking access to the deep posterior compartment. Soleus should be detached from its tibial origin proximally (beware of vessels close to soleus origin) to expose the deep posterior compartment in the proximal half of the leg. The fascia over FDL is incised, with the NV bundle (posterior tibial artery, tibial nerve) being protected in its position between tibialis posterior and soleus.

I would then check muscular viability by assessing the 4 Cs:

- Contractility
- Colour
- Consistency
- Cut (does it bleed?)

Any necrotic tissue is then excised and wounds are left open for a second look with closure/coverage at 48 hours.

5. What structures are at risk during this approach?

- Lateral: Superficial peroneal nerve
- Medial: 10 cm perforator, long saphenous vein, saphenous nerve

FURTHER READING

British Orthopaedic Association Audit Standard for Trauma (BOAST). BOAST 4: The management of severe open lower limb fractures. 2009. Accessed 1 May 2016 from https://www.boa.ac.uk/wp-content/uploads/2014/12/BOAST-4.pdf.

INDEX

A

Acetabular fossa, 84
Acetabulum fracture, 83–85
    anterior and posterior columns, 84
    classification, 85
    complications of operative treatment, 85
    management, 83, 85
    pelvis, radiograph of, 84
    radiographs, 83–84
    tear drop, 84
Achilles tendon, 215
Acromioclavicular joint injury, 115–116
    clinical assessment, 115
    management, 115–116
    radiographs, 115
Acute proximal pole fracture, 146
Advanced trauma life support (ATLS) principles,
    161–163
Age
    fracture of the distal radius and, 143, 144
    intracapsular hip fracture and, 72
    non-union and, 184
    osteoporosis and, 191
    pathological fractures and, 67
    pilon fractures and, 29
    posterior dislocation of shoulder and, 110
    triplane fractures and, 17
Airway, with cervical spine control, 161
Alcohol, 184, 191
Amputation, mangled extremity, 44–45
Anaemia, 184
Anaesthesia
    anterior shoulder dislocation, 106
    elbow dislocation, 128
    fight bite, 154
    floating knee, 56
    Galeazzi fracture, 140
    Lisfranc injury, 9
    olecranon fracture, 136
    posterior dislocation of hip, 81
    posterior dislocation of shoulder, 110
    subtalar dislocation, 12
    tibial plateau fracture, 48
    young femoral fracture, 60
Analgesia
    anterior shoulder dislocation, 106
    both bones forearm fracture, 141–142
    clavicle fracture, 113
    compartment syndrome, 37–38

    floating knee, 55
    hip fracture, 76
    ipsilateral femoral neck and shaft fracture, 64
    lunate dislocation, 152
    mangled extremity, 44
    perilunate dislocation, 148
    radial head fracture, 133
    tibial plateau fracture, 48
    young femoral fracture, 60
Angiography
    CTPA, 60
    knee dislocation, 52
    pelvic fracture, 90
Ankle, infected, *see* Infected ankle
Ankle fracture, 21–24
    classification, 21
    form of treatment, 24
    neurovascular deficit, 23
    posterior malleolus fracture, 22
    radiographs, 21, 23
    surgical outcome, 24
    syndesmosis, 24
    types, 22
Anterior approach to humerus, 197–198
    dangers, 197
    extension, 198
    indications, 197
Anterior dislocations of hip, 82
Anterior inferior tibio–fibular ligament (AITFL), 24
Anterior posterior compression (APC), pelvic
    fracture, 88
Anterior shoulder dislocation, 105–107
    history and examination, 106
    management, 106
    papers/evidence, 107
    physiotherapy, 106
    radiographs, 105–106
    recurrent instability, 106–107
Anterior superior iliac spine (ASIS), 209, 211
    dangers, 210
    extension, 210
    indications for, 209
Anterolateral approach to humerus, 199–200
    dangers of, 199
    extension, 200
    indications, 199
Antibiotics
    both bones forearm fracture, 142
    calcaneal fracture, 14

compartment syndrome, 38
damage control orthopaedics, 171
fight bite, 154
Galeazzi fracture, 140
gunshot injury, 173–174
infected ankle, 26
mangled extremity, 44
midshaft diaphyseal tibia fracture, 35
open fracture, 166
terrible triad injury, 132
tibial plateau fracture, 48
AO classification, pilon fracture, 28
Arterial injury, with knee dislocation, 52
Arteries
    dorsalis pedis, 4
    peroneal, 4
    posteror tibial, 4
Arthritis
    osteoarthritis, 24
    post-traumatic, 12, 49, 72, 85
    pre-existing knee, 48
    septic, 153, 154
    subtalar, 14
Arthroplasty
    consequences of, 72
    elbow, 124
    hip, 84
Assessment
    acromioclavicular joint injury, 115
    ATLS, 161–163
    Doppler, infected ankle, 26
    Holstein–Lewis fracture, 122
    knee dislocation, 52
    posterior dislocation of shoulder, 110
Axillary nerve, 196

B

'Bag of bones' treatment method, 124
Benefits, operative *vs.* non-operative treatment, 118
Bigelow's manoeuvre, 81
Bilateral cervical facet dislocation, 95–96
    investigation and management, 95–96
    reduction, 96
Bisphosphates for hip fracture, 66
Bisphosphonates for osteoporosis, 191, 192
Bleeding, in pelvic fracture, 88
Blood supply
    to femoral head, 71–72, 75–76
    to talus, 4
Blood tests for non-union, 185
Bohler angle, 13
Bone healing, 179
Bone lesions, mnemonics for, 69
Bone mineral density (BMD), 191
    scan, 191

Both bones forearm fracture, 141–142
    history and examination, 141–142
    radiographs, 141, 142
    surgery, 142
    treatment, 141–142
Brachioradialis, 203
Bridging, function of plate, 179–180
Buttress, function of plate, 179

C

Calcaneal fracture, 13–14, 163
    complications of surgery, 14
    management, 13–14
    mechanism of injury, 13
    nonoperative management, 14
    radiographs, 13
Calcium intake for osteoporosis, 191, 192
Cancellous screws, 177
Cefuroxime, 34–35
Cephalic vein, 196, 205
Cephalosporin, damage control orthopaedics, 171
Cerclage wires, 80
Cervical spine control, airway with, 161
Chaput fragment, with pilon fracture, 29
Chevron olecranon osteotomy, 124
Cigarette use, 191
Classification
    acetabulum fracture, 85
    acromioclavicular joint injury, 115
    ankle fracture, 21
    distal femoral fracture, 58
    Hawkins, 3
    hip fracture, 66, 75
    jersey finger, 156
    knee dislocation, 52–53
    open fracture, 167–169
    pelvic fracture, 88, 89
    perilunate dislocation, 148
    periprosthetic fracture, 79
    pilon fracture, 28–29
Clavicle fracture, 113–114
    advice, 113
    history and examination, 113
    management, 113–114
    radiographs, 113
    treatment options, 113
Clinical findings
    acromioclavicular joint injury, 115
    posterior dislocation of hip, 82
    scaphoid fracture, 145
Clinical photographs
    fight bite, 153
    infected ankle, 25
    Lisfranc injury, 8
    mangled extremity, 43

midshaft diaphyseal tibia fracture, 33–34
open fracture, 165–166
Clinical union, 184
Closed reduction
elbow dislocation, 128
lunate dislocation, 152
perilunate dislocation, 148–149
pilon fracture, 29–30
posterior dislocation of hip, 81–82
subtalar dislocation, 12
triplane fractures, 18
Comminuted fracture patterns, fixation and
replacement for, 134
Compartment syndrome, 37–39, 182
common causes, 217
development of, 166
diagnosis, 38–39, 166
fasciotomies, 38
of foot, 4
management, 38–39, 167
midshaft diaphyseal tibia fracture, 34–35
opioid analgesia for, 37–38
in pilon fractures, 28, 31
radiographs, 37
risks in, 218
Complications
acetabulum fracture, 85
calcaneal fracture, 14
ipsilateral femoral neck and shaft fracture,
64
pilon fracture, 30–31
subtalar dislocations, 12
talus fracture, 4
tibial plateau fracture, 49
Compression, function of plate, 179
Computed tomography (CT)
absence of, pelvic fracture, 88
bilateral cervical facet dislocation,
95–96
greater tuberosity fracture, 103–104
knee dislocation, 53
Lisfranc injury, 9
posterior dislocation of shoulder, 110
subtalar dislocations, 12
terrible triad injury, 132
thoracolumbar spine injury, 97
young femoral fracture, 60
Computer tomography pulmonary angiography
(CTPA), 60
Core, part of screw, 175, 176
Corona mortis, 212
Coronoid fracture, fixation, 132
Cortical screws, 176–177
Corticosteroids, 184
Cotyloid fossa, 84
Critical ischaemia, features, 58

D

Damage control orthopaedics, 171–172
management, 171–172
resuscitation, 171
Deformities
midshaft humerus fracture, 117
procurvatum, 42
proximal tibial diaphyseal fracture, 42
valgus, 42
Delayed presentation, treatment of Lisfranc
injury, 10
Delayed union, 4, 31, 142
Deltoid-splitting approach, 104
Deltopectoral approach, 195–196
dangers of, 196
extension of, 196
indications, 195
Diabetes, 184
ankle fracture and, 24
infected ankle, 24–26
Diagnosis
compartment syndrome, 37–39, 166
jersey finger, 155
Lisfranc injury, 8–9
pathological fracture, 67
scaphoid fracture, 145
young femoral fracture, 60–61
Diagnostic periteoneal lavage (DPL), 90
Die punch fragment, with pilon fracture, 29, 30
Dislocations
bilateral cervical facet, 95–96
elbow, 127–129
Galeazzi fracture, 139–140
of hip
anterior, 82
posterior, 81–82
knee, 51–53
lunate dislocation, 151–152
Monteggia fracture, 138
perilunate dislocation, 147–149
shoulder
anterior, 105–107
posterior, 109–110
subtalar, 11–12
Distal femoral fracture, 57–58
classification, 58
in emergency department, 57–58
features of critical ischaemia, 58
management, 58
radiographs, 57
Distal humerus fracture, 123–124
implants, 124
intra-articular injury, treatment, 123
radiographs, 123
surgical approach, 124

TEA for, 124
treatment choice, 124
Distal interphalangeal joint (DIPJ), 155
Distal radioulnar joint (DRUJ), 140
Distal radius, 143–144
management, 143–144
radiographs, 143, 144
Distal tibiofibular syndesmosis, diastasis at, 23
Doppler assessment, infected ankle, 26
Drill sizes, 176–177
Dual energy x-ray absorptiometry (DEXA) scan, 80, 191

E

Eikenella corrodens, 154
Elbow arthroplasty, 124
Elbow dislocation, 127–129
management, 128–129
pathoanatomy, 128
radiographs, 128
structures, damage, 128
Elderly patients
with hip fracture, 66, 76
olecranon fracture, 136
osteoporotic patient, 110
periprosthetic fracture, 79–80
with tibial plateau fractures, 48
Emergency department
acetabulum fracture, 83–85
acromioclavicular joint injury, 115–116
anterior shoulder dislocation, 105–107
ATLS principles, 161–163
bilateral cervical facet dislocation, 95–96
clavicle fracture, 113–114
compartment syndrome, 37–39
damage control orthopaedics, 171–172
distal femoral fracture in, 57–58
distal radius, 143–144
elbow dislocation, 127–129
fight bite, assessment, 153
floating knee in, 55–56
gunshot injury, 173–174
hip fracture, 65–66, 75–77
ipsilateral femoral neck and shaft fracture, 63–64
jersey finger, 155–157
lunate dislocation, 152
mangled extremity, 43–45
midshaft diaphyseal tibia fracture, 33–35
midshaft humerus fracture, 117–119
open fracture, 165–166
perilunate dislocation, 147–149
periprosthetic fracture, 79–80
pilon fracture in, 29–30
posterior dislocation of hip, 81–82

posterior dislocation of shoulder, 110
proximal humerus fracture, 101–102
radial head fracture, 133–134
terrible triad injury, 131–132
thoracolumbar spine injury, 97–98
young femoral fracture, 60
Endochondral ossification, 180
Epilepsy, posterior dislocation of shoulder and, 110
Erythema, 184
Ethnicity and osteoporosis, 191
Examination
anterior shoulder dislocation, 106
both bones forearm fracture, 141–142
clavicle fracture, 113
Holstein–Lewis fracture, 122
infected ankle, 26
midshaft humerus fracture, 117
pelvic fracture, 87
radial head fracture, 133
Exchange nailing, 185; *see also* Non-union of diaphyseal fractures of tibia
Extensor digitorum brevis, 4
Extraperitoneal rupture, 90

F

Fasciotomies, compartment syndrome, 38
Fat emboli, 182
Fat embolus syndrome, 60–61
Femoral fracture, 188
Femoral head, blood supply to, 71–72, 75–76
Fever, 184
Fibular fracture, with pilon fracture, 30
Fight bites, 153–154
assessment, in emergency department, 153
clinical photograph, 153
operative management, 154
Fixation
Monteggia fracture, 138
tension band wire and plate fixation, selection, 135
terrible triad injury, 132
Flaps, for soft tissue coverage, 167
Flexor digitorum profundus (FDP) muscle, 155
Flexor digitorum superficialis (FDS), 155
Flexor hallucis longus (FHL), 215
Floating knee, 55–56
management in emergency department, 55–56
radiographs, 55
Flutes, part of screw, 175, 176
Focused assessment with sonography for trauma (FAST) scans, 90
Fracture factors in non-union, 184
Fracture Risk Assessment Tool (FRAX), 191
Functional bracing, 118

G

Galeazzi fracture, 139–140
    isolated diaphyseal fracture of radius, 140
    management, 140
    radiographs, 139–140
    stabilisers of distal radioulnar joint, 140
Garden classification, hip fracture, 75
Gilula lines, lunate dislocation, 151
Gissane angle, 13
Grade, open fracture, 167–168
Greater tuberosity fracture, 103–104
    degree of displacement, 104
    management, 103–104
    radiographs, 103
Gunshot injury, 173–174
    management, 173–174
    radiographs, 173–174
Gustilo–Anderson classification system, for open
       fractures, 167–168

H

Haematoma
    bone healing, stage, 180
    tamponade effect of, 72
Haematuria, presence of, 90
Haemorrhage
    control, 161–162
    damage control orthopaedics, 171
    mangled extremity, 43–44
    resuscitation, in pelvic fracture, 90
Hard callus, stage of bone healing, 180
Hawkins classification, talus fracture, 3
Hawkins sign, 5
Head, part of screw, 175, 176
Hemiarthroplasty, 76, 124
Henry's approach to the forearm, 203–205
Heterotopic ossification, 85
Hip, dislocation of
    anterior, 82
    posterior, 81–82
Hip fracture, 65–66, 75–77
    blood supply to femoral head, 75–76
    chest radiograph, 76
    classification, 66, 75
    examination and investigations, 76
    fragments, position, 65
    information, from history, 76
    intracapsular, young patient, 71–73
    investigations, 66
    management, 66, 76–77
    radiographs, 65, 75
Holstein–Lewis fracture, 121–122
    assessment, 122
    history and examination, 122
    pattern, problems with, 121–122
    radiographs, 121
    surgical management, 122
Hormone replacement therapy, 191
Humeral osteotomies, 197
Humerus
    anterior approach to, 197–198
    anterolateral approach to, 199–200
    Kocher's approach to, 207–208
    posterior approach to distal, 201–202
Humerus fracture
    distal, 123–124
    midshaft, 117–119
    proximal, 99–102, 101–102
Hyperparathyroidism, 184
Hypothyroidism, 184

I

Ilioinguinal approach, 211–213
    indications, 211
    risk, 213
Ilioinguinal nerve, 211
Ilizarov Spatial Frame fixation, 48
IM, *see* Intramedullary (IM) nailing
Imaging
    Lisfranc injury, 8–9
    lunate dislocation, 151
    subtalar dislocation, 11, 12
Implants
    distal humerus fracture, 124
    intramedullary, 66
    radial head, 132
    terrible triad injury, 132
Indications, for operative intervention
    clavicle fracture, 114
    fixing, posterior dislocation of hip, 82
    midshaft humerus fracture, 118
    proximal humerus fracture, 100
    radial head fracture, 133–134
    scaphoid fracture, 146
    thoracolumbar spine injury, 97–98
Infected ankle, 25–26
    clinical photograph, 25
    management, 26
    management, in outpatient clinic, 25–26
Inflammation, stage of bone healing, 180
Information, from history, 76
Internervous plane utilisation
    in anterior (brachialis splitting) approach, 197
    in anterolateral approach to humerus, 199,
       200
    in deltopectoral approach, 195
    in ilioinguinal approach, 211
    in Kocher's approach to humerus, 207, 208
    in pilon fracture, 30

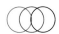

in posterior approach to humerus, 201
in posterolateral approach to ankle, 215
in Smith–Petersen approach, 209, 210
in volar approach to forearm, 203
Intra-articular displacement, fractures with, 18
Intra-articular fragments, with pilon fracture, 29
Intra-articular injury, treatment, 123
Intracapsular hip fracture young patient, 71–73
    blood supply to femoral head, 71–72
    closed reduction, 72
    limitations, 72–73
    management, 72–73
    radiographs, 71
    treatment options, 72–73
Intramedullary nail, 183
Intramedullary (IM) nailing
    bone healing, 179
    compartment syndrome, 37, 38–39
    damage control orthopaedics, 172
    floating knee, 56
    gunshot injury, 173
    hip fracture, 66
    ipsilateral femoral neck and shaft fracture, 64
    locking bolt and, 176
    midshaft diaphyseal tibia fracture, 35
    open fracture, 166
    tibial diaphyseal fracture, 42
Intraosseous blood supply, 72
Intraperitoneal rupture, 90
Investigations
    bilateral cervical facet dislocation, 95–96
    hip fracture, 66, 76
    ipsilateral femoral neck and shaft fracture, 64
    knee dislocation, 53
    midshaft diaphyseal tibia fracture, 34–35
    periprosthetic fracture, 79–80
    pilon fracture, 28
    posterior dislocation of shoulder, 110
    thoracolumbar spine injury, 97
    tibial plateau fracture, 48
Ipsilateral femoral neck and shaft fracture, 63–64
    complications, 64
    investigation, 64
    management, 64
    operative plan for, 64
    radiographs, 63
    surgery, sequence of, 64
Isolated diaphyseal fracture of radius, Galeazzi
    fracture, 140

J

Jersey finger, 155–157
    classification, 156
    diagnosis, 155
    management, 156–157

Journal of Bone and Joint Surgery, 168
Judet classification, acetabulum fracture, 85

K

Kirschner wires, 144
Knee dislocation, 51–53
    arterial injury, 52
    assessment, 52
    classification, 52–53
    investigation and management, 53
    management, 52, 53
    peroneal nerve injury, 53
    popliteal artery at particular risk of injury, 52
    radiographs, 51–52
Kocher–Langenbeck approach, 82
Kocher's approach to the humerus, 207–208
    dangers, 207
    differences from Kaplan's interval, 208
    indications, 207
K-wires
    calcaneal fracture, 14
    Galeazzi fracture, 140
    intracapsular hip fracture, 72
    jersey finger, fracture repair, 157
    Lisfranc injury, 9, 10
    lunate dislocation, 152
    perilunate dislocation, 149
    pilon fracture, 30
    talus fracture, 4
    tibial diaphyseal fracture, 42

L

Lag screws, 176–177, 179
Lateral collateral ligament (LCL), 128
Lateral compression (LC), pelvic fracture, 88
Lateral starting point, 42
Lauge–Hansen classification, ankle fracture, 21,
    22
LEAP (Lower Extremity Assessment Project)
    study, 44, 166
Leg fasciotomy, 217–218
Length, of screws, 177
Letournel classification, acetabulum fracture, 85
Limb salvage, mangled extremity, 44
Limitations, intracapsular hip fracture young
    patient, 72–73
Lisfranc injury, 7–10
    clinical photograph, 8
    computed tomography, 9
    delayed presentation, 10
    diagnosis, 8–9
    imaging, 8–9
    management, 9–10
    radiographs, 8, 9

Locking bolt with IM nail, screws, 176
Loss of appetite, 184
Lower Extremity Assessment Project (LEAP)
    study, 44, 166
Lower limb and pelvic trauma
  acetabulum fracture, 83–85
  ankle fracture, 21–24
  calcaneal fracture, 13–14
  compartment syndrome, 37–39
  distal femoral fracture, 57–58
  floating knee, 55–56
  hip fracture, 65–66, 75–77
  infected ankle, 25–26
  ipsilateral femoral neck and shaft fracture,
    63–64
  knee dislocation, 51–53
  Lisfranc injury, 7–10
  mangled extremity, 43–45
  midshaft diaphyseal tibia fracture, 33–35
  pathological fracture, 67–69
  pelvic fracture, 87–91
  periprosthetic fracture, 79–80
  pilon fracture, 27–31
  posterior dislocation of hip, 81–82
  subtalar dislocation, 11–12
  talus fracture, 3–5
  tibial diaphyseal fracture (proximal), 41–42
  tibial plateau fracture, 47–49
  triplane fractures, 17–19
  young femoral fracture, 59–61
Lunate dislocation, 151–152
  Gilula lines, 151
  management, 152
  radiographs, 151
Lunotriquetral ligament, 149

M

Magnetic resonance imaging (MRI)
  bilateral cervical facet dislocation, 96
  knee dislocation, 53
  thoracolumbar spine injury, 97
Malnutrition, 184
Malreduction, of ulna, 138
Mal-union, 4, 30, 31, 42, 102, 142
Management
  acetabular fractures, 211
  acetabulum fracture, 83, 85
  acromioclavicular joint injury, 115–116
  ankle fracture, 24
  anterior shoulder dislocation, 106
  bilateral cervical facet dislocation, 95–96
  both bones forearm fracture, 141–142
  calcaneal fracture, 13–14
  clavicle fracture, 113–114
  compartment syndrome, 38–39, 167

damage control orthopaedics, 171–172
distal femoral fracture, 58
distal humerus fracture, 123, 124
distal radius, 143–144
elbow dislocation, 128–129
fight bite, 154
floating knee, 55–56
Galeazzi fracture, 140
greater tuberosity fracture, 103–104
gunshot injury, 173–174
hip fracture, 66, 76–77
Holstein–Lewis fracture, 122
infected ankle, 26
injury, ATLS principles, 161–163
intracapsular hip fracture young patient,
    72–73
ipsilateral femoral neck and shaft fracture,
    64
jersey finger, 156–157
knee dislocation, 52, 53
Lisfranc injury, 9–10
lunate dislocation, 152
mangled extremity, 43–44
midshaft diaphyseal tibia fracture, 34–35
midshaft humerus fracture, 117
Monteggia fracture, 138
non-accidental injury, 188
olecranon fracture, 135–136
open fracture, 165–166
osteoporosis, 191
pelvic fracture, 87, 89–90
perilunate dislocation, 148–149
periprosthetic fracture, 79–80
pilon fracture, 28, 29–31
posterior dislocation of hip, 81–82
posterior dislocation of shoulder, 110
principles, pathological fracture and, 68
proximal humerus fracture, 100, 102
radial head fracture, 133
scaphoid fracture, 145–146
subtalar dislocation, 11–12
talus fracture, 3–4
terrible triad injury, 131–132
thoracolumbar spine injury, 97
tibial diaphyseal fracture (proximal), 42
tibial plateau fracture, 48
triplane fractures, 17–18
urethral injury, pelvic fracture and, 89–90
young femoral fracture, 60–61
Mangled extremity, 43–45
  amputation, 44–45
  clinical photograph, 43
  guidance from BOA and BAPRAS, 44–45
  limb salvage, 44
  management, 43–44
  radiographs, 44

MCFA (medial circumflex femoral artery), 75, 82
Mechanism of injury
    calcaneal fracture, 13
    pilon fracture, 28
    posterior dislocation of hip, 82
    talus fracture, 3
Medial circumflex femoral artery (MCFA), 75, 82
Medial collateral ligament (MCL), 128–129
Medial malleolus, with pilon fracture, 29
Medial plantar ecchymosis, 8
'Mercedes Benz' sign, 24
Microbiology examination, infected ankle, 26
Midshaft diaphyseal humerus fracture, 118
Midshaft diaphyseal tibia fracture, 33–35
    investigation, 34–35
    management, 34–35
    radiographs and clinical photographs, 33–34
Midshaft humerus fracture, 117–119
    examination, 117
    history, 117
    indications for operative treatment, 118
    management, 117
    neurology and vascular status, reassessing, 118
    radial nerve symptoms, 118
    radiographs, 117
    residual displacement/deformity, 117
    risks and benefits of operative *vs.*
        non-operative treatment, 118
    Sarmiento functional brace, 118
Mirels score, 68
Monteggia fracture, 137–138
    management, 138
    radiographs, 137–138
    ulna with plate fixation, 138
Morel–Lavallée lesion, 83, 85, 87
Muscular viability, 218
Musculocutaneous nerve, 196, 198

N

Nailing
    anterograde and retrograde, 56
    intramedullary, *see* Intramedullary (IM) nailing
    semi-extended, 42
Nails and external fixators, 181–182
National Institute for Health and Clinical
        Excellence (NICE) guidelines, 66
Neurapraxia, 121
Neurogenic shock, 98
Neurologic deficit, bilateral cervical facet
        dislocation, 96
Neurovascular deficit
    ankle fracture, 23
    distal radius, 143

radial head fracture, 133
    tibial plateau fracture, 48
Neurovascularly intact injury, pilon fracture, 29–30
Neutralisation, function of plate, 179
NICE guidance, 191
Non-accidental injury, 187–189
    features of, 188
    managing patient and family during, 188
    relevant literature, 188–189
Non-ambulatory children, 188
Nonoperative management, calcaneal fracture, 14
Non-responder to resuscitation, pelvic fracture, 90
Non-union, 4, 26, 31, 102, 118, 142, 146
Non-union of diaphyseal fractures of tibia, 183–185
    atrophic, 184
    clinical findings in, 184
    definition, 183
    diagnosis, 183
    factors causing, 184
    hypertrophic, 184
    surgery, principles of, 185
    types of, 184
NSAIDs, 184

O

Oestrogen receptor modulators
    for osteoporosis, 192
Olecranon fracture, 135–136
    alternative treatment, 135
    co-morbidities and anaesthetic risks, 136
    management, 135, 136
    plate fixation, selection, 135
    radiographs, 135
    tension band wire fixation
        principle, 135
        selection, 135
Olecranon osteotomy, 124
Open fracture, 165–169
    classification, 167–169
    clinical photograph, 165–166
    grade, 167–168
    initial management, 165–166
    postoperative period, 166–167
    soft tissue coverage, 167, 168
    surgery, 166
Operative plan, for ipsilateral femoral neck and
        shaft fracture, 64
Opioid analgesia, compartment syndrome, 37–38
Orthopaedics, damage control, 171–172
Osteoarthritis, 24

Osteomyelitis, 31, 153
Osteopenia, 191–192
Osteoporosis, 110, 144, 176, 177, 191–192
    DEXA scan, 191
    risk factors, 191
    treatment of, 192
Osteotomy, chevron olecranon, 124
Outcomes
    for injury and treatment, subtalar
        dislocations, 12
    surgical, ankle fracture, 24
Ovarian failure, 191

P

Paediatric fractures, 184
Pain, compartment syndrome, 38
Palmar carpal tunnel approach, 152
Partial responder to resuscitation, pelvic
    fracture, 90
Pathoanatomy, of elbow dislocation, 128
Pathological fracture, 67–69
    differential diagnosis, 67
    intracapsular hip fracture young patient,
        71–73
    management principles and, 68
    radiographs, 67–68
Patient factors in non-union, 184
Patient positioning, *see* Positioning, patient
Patients, classification, 90
Pauwels hip fractures, 64
Pelvic fracture, 87–91
    classification, 88, 89
    CT, absence of, 88
    examination, 87
    management, 87, 89–90
    radiographs, 87, 88, 89
    responses to resuscitation, 90
    retrograde urethrogram, 91
    sources of bleeding in, 88
    urethral injury, 89–90
    urological injury, signs, 89–90
Perilunate dislocation, 147–149
    classification, 148
    management, 148–149
    radiographs, 147–148
Peripheral vascular disease, 184
Periprosthetic fracture, 79–80
    classification, 79
    management and investigation, 79–80
    radiographs, 79
    treatment options, 80
Peroneal nerve injury, knee dislocation and, 53
Physeal fractures, 17
Physiotherapy, for shoulder rehabilitation, 106
Pilon fracture, 27–31

classification, 28–29
closed reduction, 29–30
complications, 30–31
fibular fracture with, 30
intra-articular fragments with, 29
investigations, 28
management, 28, 29–31
mechanism of injury, 28
neurovascularly intact injury, 29–30
radiographs, 27–28
reducing and fixing, 30
Pin tract infection, 49
Pitch, part of screw, 175, 176
Plate fixation
    Monteggia fracture, 138
    for olecranon fracture, 135
Plates, 179–180
    bone healing, lag screw and neutralisation
        plate, 179
    functions
        bridging, 179–180
        buttress, 179
        compression, 179
        neutralisation, 179
        tension band, 179
    strength, 179
Poller blocking screws, 42
Popliteal artery, at particular risk of injury, 52
Positioning, patient
    in anterior (brachialis splitting) approach, 197
    in anterolateral approach to humerus, 199
    in deltopectoral approach, 195
    floating knee, 56
    in ilioinguinal approach, 211
    in Kocher's approach to humerus, 207
    in posterior approach to humerus, 201
    in posterolateral approach to ankle, 215
    in Smith–Petersen approach, 209
    tibial plateau fracture, 48–49
    in volar approach to forearm, 203
Posterior approach to distal humerus, 201–202
    dangers of, 201–202
    extension, 202
    indications, 201
Posterior dislocation, of hip, 81–82
    clinical and radiographic findings, 82
    closed reduction, 81–82
    indications for fixing, 82
    management, 81–82
    mechanism of injury, 82
    posterior wall fracture, fixing, 82
    postoperative management, 82
    radiographs, 81
Posterior dislocation of shoulder, 109–110
    investigation and assessment, 110
    management, 110

radiographs, 110
reconstructive options, 110
Posterior inferior tibio–fibular ligament (PITFL), 24
Posterior interosseus nerve (PIN), 204, 205, 208
Posterior malleolus fracture, 22
Posterolateral approach to ankle, 215
dangers, 215
indications, 215
Post-menopausal women, 191
Postoperative period
open fracture, 166–167
posterior dislocation of hip, 82
Post-traumatic arthritis, 12, 49, 72, 85
Premature menopause, 191
Pressure monitoring
arterial, 166
continuous, 166
Principles, trauma
ATLS, 161–163
damage control orthopaedics, 171–172
gunshot injury, 173–174
open fracture, 165–169
plates, 179–180
screws, 175–177
Procurvatum deformity, 42
Profunda brachii, 202
Pronation–abduction (PAB) type ankle fracture, 22
Pronation–external rotation (PER) type ankle fracture, 22
Pronation injuries, 22
Proximal humerus fracture, 99–102
indications, operative intervention, 100
management, 100, 102
radiographs, 99, 101
surgery, 102
Proximal interphalangeal joint (PIPJ), 155
Proximal tibial diaphyseal fracture, 41–42
Pullout strength, of screws, 176
Pulmonary complications, 182

R

Radial artery, 205
Radial head fracture, 133–134
fixation and replacement for comminuted fracture types, 134
history and examination, 133
indications for surgery, 133–134
management, 133
radiographs, 133
Radial nerve fibres, 197
superficial, 204
Radial nerve palsy, 121
Radial nerve symptoms, 118

Radiographic union, 184
Radiographs
acetabulum fracture, 83–84
acromioclavicular joint injury, 115
ankle fracture, 21, 23
anterior shoulder dislocation, 105–106
both bones forearm fracture, 141, 142
calcaneal fracture, 13
clavicle fracture, 113
compartment syndrome, 37
distal femoral fracture, 57
distal humerus fracture, 123
distal radius, 143, 144
elbow dislocation, 128
floating knee, 55
Galeazzi fracture, 139–140
greater tuberosity fracture, 103
gunshot injury, 173–174
hip fracture (subtrochanteric region), 65, 75
Holstein–Lewis fracture, 121
infected ankle, 26
intracapsular hip fracture young patient, 71
ipsilateral femoral neck and shaft fracture, 63
knee dislocation, 51–52
Lisfranc injury, 8, 9
lunate dislocation, 151
mangled extremity, 44
midshaft diaphyseal tibia fracture, 33–34
midshaft humerus fracture, 117
monteggia fracture, 137–138
olecranon fracture, 135
pathological fracture, 67–68
pelvic fracture, 84, 87, 88, 89
perilunate dislocation, 147–148
periprosthetic fracture, 79
pilon fracture, 27–28
posterior dislocation of hip, 81, 82
posterior dislocation of shoulder, 110
proximal humerus fracture, 99, 101
radial head fracture, 133
scaphoid fracture, 145
subtalar dislocation, 11
talus fracture, 3
terrible triad injury, 131
tibial diaphyseal fracture, 41–42
tibial plateau fracture, 47
triplane fracture, 17–19
young femoral fracture, 59–60
Radius, isolated diaphyseal fracture of, 140
Raloxifene for osteoporosis, 192
Reamed nails, 181–182
Reconstruction, posterior dislocation of shoulder, 110
Recurrent instability, anterior shoulder dislocation, 106–107

Reduction
    bilateral cervical facet dislocation, 96
    elbow dislocation, 128
    intracapsular hip fracture young patient, 72
    lunate dislocation, 152
    Monteggia fracture, 138
    perilunate dislocation, 148–149
    pilon fracture, 30
    posterior dislocation of hip, 81–82
    subtalar dislocation, 12
    triplane fractures, 18
Remodelling, stage of bone healing, 180
Replacement
    for comminuted fracture types, 134
    elbow, 124
    fluid (blood), 90
    hip, 72, 76, 79, 80
    intracapsular hip fracture, 72
    periprosthetic fracture, 79, 80
    radial head, 131, 132, 134
    terrible triad injury, 131, 132
Residual displacement, midshaft humerus
            fracture, 117
Respiratory distress, 161
Responses to resuscitation, pelvic fracture and, 90
Resuscitation
    damage control orthopaedics, 171
    responses to, pelvic fracture, 90
Retrograde urethrogram, pelvic fracture, 91
Rigidity/stiffness of nail, 181
Rigors, 184
Risks
    anaesthetic, olecranon fracture, 136
    operative *vs.* non-operative treatment, 118
Rockwood system of classification,
            acromioclavicular joint injury, 115
Rotational thromboelastometry (ROTEM), 162
Ruedi and Allgower classification, pilon fracture,
            28–29
Russell–Taylor classification, hip fracture, 66

S

Sarmiento functional brace, 118
Scandinavian Sarcoma Group, 68
Scaphoid fracture, 145–146
    acute proximal pole fracture, 146
    clinical examination, 145
    diagnosis, 145
    indications for acute fixation of, 146
    management, 145–146
    radiographs, 145
    surgery, 145–146
    undisplaced scaphoid waist fracture, 145–146
Scapholunate ligament, 148, 149
Scapular fractures, 163

Scoring system
    mangled extremity, 44
    pathological fracture, 68
Screws, 175–177
    cancellous screws, 177
    cortical, 176–177
    different parts, 175–176
    drill sizes, 176–177
    function, 175
    function of parts, 176
    lag, 176–177, 179
    lag screws, 176–177
    locking bolt with intramedullary nail, 176
    small and large fragment cortical screw, 176–177
    tensile strength *vs.* pullout strength, 176
    type, 176
    working length, 177
Seizure, 110
Self-tapping screws, 177
Sepsis, signs of, 25
Septic arthritis, 153, 154
Shoulder dislocation
    anterior, 105–107
    posterior, 109–110
Signpost injuries, 162–163
Sliding hip screw device, 72
Smith–Petersen approach, 64, 209–210
Smoking, 14
Soft callus, stage of bone healing, 180
Soft tissue coverage, open fracture, 167, 168
Soft tissue swelling, 14
Spinal fractures, 162
Spinal shock, 98
Spine and upper limb trauma
    acromioclavicular joint injury, 115–116
    anterior shoulder dislocation, 105–107
    bilateral cervical facet dislocation, 95–96
    both bones forearm fracture, 141–142
    clavicle fracture, 113–114
    distal humerus fracture, 123–124
    distal radius, 143–144
    elbow dislocation, 127–129
    fight bite, 153–154
    Galeazzi fracture, 139–140
    greater tuberosity fracture, 103–104
    Holstein–Lewis fracture, 121–122
    jersey finger, 155–157
    lunate dislocation, 151–152
    midshaft humerus fracture, 117–119
    Monteggia fracture, 137–138
    olecranon fracture, 135–136
    perilunate dislocation, 147–149
    posterior dislocation of shoulder, 109–110
    proximal humerus fracture, 99–100,
            101–102
    radial head fracture, 133–134

Index

scaphoid fracture, 145–146
terrible triad injury, 131–132
thoracolumbar spine injury, 97–98
Split-thickness skin graft (STSG), 167
Spur sign, 85
Stabilisers, of distal radioulnar joint, 140
Staphylococcus aureus, 154
Steinmann Pin, 14, 42
Sternal fractures, 163
Steroids, 191
Strength, plates, 179
Strontium ranelate
for osteoporosis, 192
Subtalar dislocations, 11–12
closed reduction, 12
complications, 12
initial management, 11
outcome for injury and treatment, 12
plan for definitive management, 12
radiographs, 11
Subtrochanteric region (hip fracture), 65–66
classification, 66
fragments, position, 65
investigations, 66
management, 66
radiographs, 65
Superficial peroneal nerve (SPN), 217
Supination–adduction (SAD) type injury, 21,
22
Supination–external rotation (SER) type ankle
fracture, 22
Sural nerve, 215
Surgery
ankle fracture, 24
both bones forearm fracture, 142
calcaneal fracture, 13–14
distal femoral fracture, 58
distal humerus fracture, 124
floating knee, 56
Holstein–Lewis fracture, 122
ipsilateral femoral neck and shaft fracture,
64
midshaft diaphyseal tibia fracture, 35
open fracture, 166
pathological fracture, 68
pilon fracture, 29–30
posterior dislocation of hip, 82
proximal humerus fracture, 102
radial head fracture, 133–134
scaphoid fracture, 145–146
thoracolumbar spine injury, 97–98
tibial plateau fracture, 48–49
Surgical factors in non-union, 184
Sweats, 184
Symmetrical chest wall movement, 161
Syndesmosis injury, ankle fracture, 24

T
Talus fracture, 3–5
blood supply, 4
classification system, 3
complications, 4
Hawkins sign, 5
injury
management, 3–4
mechanism of, 3
radiography, 3
Tarsometatarsal (TMT) joints, 8, 9
Taylor Spatial Frame fixation, 48
Tear drop, pelvic, 84
Tensile strength, of screws, 176
Tension band
function of plate, 179
wire fixation, for olecranon fracture
principle, 135
selection, 135
Terrible triad injury, 131–132
operative sequence for fixation and repair,
132
radiographs, 131
treatment, 131–132
Tetanus immunoglobulin, gunshot injury, 173
Tetanus toxoid, mangled extremity, 44
Thigh tourniquet, 9, 14, 30, 44, 48
Thoracolumbar Injury Classification and
Severity Score (TLICS), 97–98
Thoracolumbar spinal orthosis (TLSO), 97
Thoracolumbar spine injury, 97–98
indications for surgery, 97–98
investigation and management, 97
neurogenic shock and spinal shock, 98
Threads, part of screw, 176
Tibia fracture, midshaft diaphyseal, 33–35
Tibial diaphyseal fracture (proximal), 41–42
deformities, responsibility, 42
management, 42
radiographs, 41–42
Tibial plateau fracture, 47–49
complications, 49
investigation, 48
management, 48
patient positioning and surgical approach,
48–49
radiographs, 47
treatment options, 48
weight bearing status/restrictions, 49
Tibial shaft fracture, 183
Tillaux fractures, triplane *vs.*, 19
Torsional stiffness, 181
Total elbow replacement (TEA), for distal
humerus fractures, 124
Tranexamic acid, 162

Trauma
    general principles
        ATLS, 161–163
        damage control orthopaedics, 171–172
        gunshot injury, 173–174
        open fracture, 165–169
        plates, 179–180
        screws, 175–177
    lower limb and pelvic, *see* Lower limb and
        pelvic trauma
    spine and upper limb, *see* Spine and upper
        limb trauma
Triangular fibrocartilaginous complex (TFCC), 140
Triplane fractures, 17–19
    age, 17
    closed reduction, 18
    describing, 17
    management, 17–18
    radiographs, 17–19
    Tillaux *vs.*, 19
    zone of physis, 17
T-score, 191
Tug test, 166
Tumour biopsies/resections, 197

U

Ulna, malreduction of, 138
Ulnar nerve, 202
Undisplaced scaphoid waist fracture, 145–146
Unreamed nails, 181–182
Urethral catheterisation, 89–90
Urethral injury, pelvic fracture and, 89–90
Urological injury, signs, 89–90
Urological trauma, 87

V

Valgus deformity, 42
Vancouver system of classification,
    periprosthetic fracture, 79
Vascular injuries, with knee dislocation, 52
Velcro straps, 118
Vitamin D, supplementary, 69
    for osteoporosis, 191, 192
Volar approach to the forearm, 203–205
    dangers of, 204–205
    extension, 205
    indications, 203
Volkmann fragment, with pilon fracture, 29

W

Watson–Jones approach, 72
Weaver–Dunn procedure, 115
Weightbearing status/restrictions, tibial plateau
    fracture, 49
Weight loss, 184
Wires
    cerclage, 80
    Kirschner, 144
    K-wires, *see* K-wires
    tension band wire fixation, for olecranon
        fracture, 135
Wolff's law, 180
Working length, 181
    of screws, 177
Wrinkle test, 14
Wrist drop, 118

X

X-rays
    anterior shoulder dislocation, 105–106
    elbow dislocation, 128–129
    pelvic fracture, 88

Y

Young and Burgess classification, of pelvic
    fractures, 88, 89
Young femoral fracture, 59–61
    differential diagnosis, 60–61
    in emergency department, 60
    management, 60–61
    procedure, 60
    radiographs, 59–60
Young patient, intracapsular hip fracture,
    71–73
    blood supply to femoral head, 71–72
    closed reduction, 72
    limitations, 72–73
    management, 72–73
    radiographs, 71
    treatment options, 72–73

Z

Zone of physis, triplane fractures, 17
Z-score, 191